# MAKING SENSE of the ECG

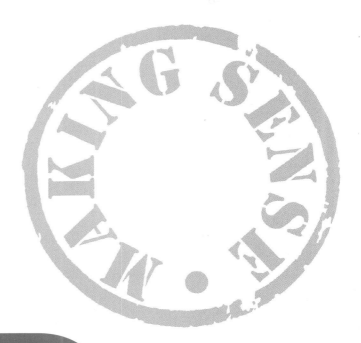

# MAKING SENSE of the
# ECG

## A hands-on guide

## Fourth edition

Andrew R Houghton
Consultant Cardiologist, Grantham and District Hospital
and Visiting Fellow, University of Lincoln,
Lincolnshire, UK

David Gray
formerly Reader in Medicine and Honorary Consultant Physician,
Department of Cardiovascular Medicine,
University Hospital,
Queen's Medical Centre,
Nottingham, UK

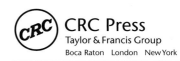

**CRC Press**
Taylor & Francis Group
Boca Raton   London   New York

CRC Press is an imprint of the
Taylor & Francis Group, an **informa** business

CRC Press
Taylor & Francis Group
6000 Broken Sound Parkway NW, Suite 300
Boca Raton, FL 33487-2742

© 2014 by Taylor & Francis Group, LLC
CRC Press is an imprint of Taylor & Francis Group, an Informa business

Printed on acid-free paper
Version Date: 20131203

Printed and bound in India by Replika Press Pvt. Ltd.

International Standard Book Number-13: 978-1-4441-8182-1 (Paperback)

### Library of Congress Cataloging-in-Publication Data

Houghton, Andrew R., author.
  Making sense of the ECG : a hands-on guide / Andrew Houghton, David Gray. -- Fourth edition.
    p. ; cm. -- (Making sense of)
  Includes bibliographical references and index.
  ISBN 978-1-4441-8182-1 (pbk. : alk. paper)
  I. Gray, David, 1949- author. II. Title. III. Series: Making sense (Boca Raton, Fla.)
  [DNLM: 1. Electrocardiography--Handbooks. 2. Heart Diseases--diagnosis--Handbooks. WG 39]

RC683.5.E5
616.1'207547--dc23                                                                                    2013045994

**Visit the Taylor & Francis Web site at**
**http://www.taylorandfrancis.com**

**and the CRC Press Web site at**
**http://www.crcpress.com**

*To Kathryn and Caroline*

# Contents

# Preface to the fourth edition

The primary aim of this fourth edition of *Making Sense of the ECG* remains the same as all its predecessors – to provide the reader with a comprehensive yet readable introduction to ECG interpretation, supplemented by clinical information about how to act upon your findings.

We have substantially restructured the text for this new edition, breaking down the rhythm section into several new chapters to make this important topic easier to understand while providing additional detail. The section on how to perform an ECG recording has been substantially expanded, and we have added new chapters on cardiac anatomy and physiology, and also on ECG reporting. The text has been updated throughout to incorporate the latest clinical guidelines, and suggestions for further reading now feature at the end of every chapter.

The larger format of this edition has given us the opportunity to improve the ECGs, many of which are presented in their full 12-lead format for the first time. Our companion volume, *Making Sense of the ECG: Cases for Self-Assessment*, has also been fully revised and updated to ensure that both books interweave seamlessly for those wishing to assess their learning.

Once again, we are grateful to everyone who has taken the time to comment on the text and to provide us with ECGs from their collections. Finally, we would like to thank all the staff at CRC Press who have contributed to the success of the *Making Sense* series of books.

**Andrew R Houghton**
**David Gray**
*2014*

# Acknowledgements

We would like to thank everyone who gave us suggestions and constructive criticism while we prepared each edition of *Making Sense of the ECG*. We are particularly grateful to the following for their invaluable comments on the text and for allowing us to use ECGs from their collections:

Mookhter Ajij
Khin Maung Aye
Stephanie Baker
Michael Bamber
Muneer Ahmad Bhat
Gabriella Captur
Andrea Charman
Nigel Dewey
Matthew Donnelly
Ian Ferrer
Catherine Goult
Lawrence Green
Mahesh Harishchandra

Michael Holmes
Safiy Karim
Dave Kendall
Jeffrey Khoo
Daniel Law
Diane Lunn
Iain Lyburn
Sonia Lyburn
Martin Melville
Cara Mercer
Yuji Murakawa
Francis Murgatroyd
V B S Naidu

Vicky Nelmes
Claire Poole
George B Pradhan
Jane Robinson
Catherine Scott
Penelope R Sensky
Neville Smith
Gary Spiers
Andrew Staniforth
Andrew Stein
Robin Touquet
Upul Wijayawardhana
Bernadette Williamson

We are also grateful to the Resuscitation Council (UK) for their permission to reproduce algorithms from their adult Advanced Life Support guidelines (2010).

Finally, we would also like to express our gratitude to Dr Joanna Koster and the rest of the publishing team at CRC Press for their encouragement, guidance and support during this project.

# CHAPTER 1

# Anatomy and physiology

The heart is a hollow muscular organ that pumps blood around the body. With each beat, it pumps, at rest, about 70 millilitres of blood and considerably more during exercise. Over a 70-year life span and at a rate of around 70 beats per minute, the heart will beat over 2.5 billion times.

The heart consists of four main chambers (left and right atria, and left and right ventricles) and four valves (aortic, mitral, pulmonary and tricuspid). Venous blood returns to the right atrium via the superior and inferior vena cavae, and leaves the right ventricle for the lungs via the pulmonary artery. Oxygenated blood from the lungs returns to the left atrium via the four pulmonary veins, and leaves the left ventricle via the aorta (Fig. 1.1).

The heart is made up of highly specialized cardiac muscle comprising myocardial cells (**myocytes**), which differs markedly from skeletal muscle because heart muscle:

- is under the control of the autonomic nervous system
- contracts in a repetitive and rhythmic manner
- has a large number of mitochondria which make the myocytes resistant to fatigue
- cannot function adequately in anaerobic (ischaemic) conditions.

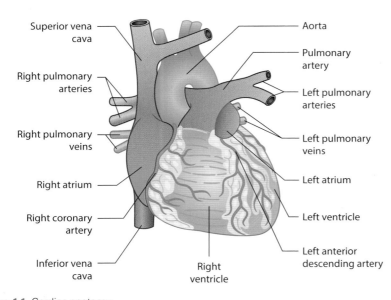

**Figure 1.1** Cardiac anatomy.

Key point:  • The heart and major vessels.

## CARDIAC ACTIVATION

Myocytes are essentially contractile but are capable of generating and transmitting electrical activity. Myocytes are interconnected by cytoplasmic bridges or syncytia, so once one myocyte cell membrane is activated (depolarized), a wave of depolarization spreads rapidly to adjacent cells.

Myocardial cells are capable of being:

- **pacemaker cells** – these are found primarily in the sinoatrial (SA) node and produce a spontaneous electrical discharge
- **conducting cells** – these are found in:
  - the atrioventricular (AV) node
  - the bundle of His and bundle branches
  - the Purkinje fibres
- **contractile cells** – these form the main cell type in the atria and ventricles.

All myocytes are self-excitable with their own intrinsic contractile rhythm. Cardiac cells in the SA node located high up in the right atrium generate action potentials or impulses at a rate of about 60–100 per minute, a slightly faster rate than cells elsewhere such as the AV node (typically 40–60 per minute) or the ventricular conducting system (30–40 per minute), so the SA node becomes the heart pacemaker, dictating the rate and timing of action potentials that trigger cardiac contraction, overriding the potential of other cells to generate impulses. However, should the SA node fail, or an impulse not reach the ventricles, cardiac contraction may be initiated by these secondary sites ('escape rhythms', p. 102).

('escape rhythms', p. 102).

### THE CARDIAC ACTION POTENTIAL

The process of triggering cardiac cells into function is called *cardiac excitation-contraction coupling*. Cells remain in a resting state until activated by changes in voltage due to the complex movement of sodium, potassium and calcium across the cell membrane (Fig. 1.2); these are similar to changes which occur in nerve cells.

**Phase 4:** At rest, there is little spontaneous depolarization as the $Na^+/K^+/ATPase$ pump maintains a negative stable resting membrane potential of about –90 mV. Some cardiac cells display automaticity or spontaneous regular action potentials, which generates action potentials in adjacent cells linked by cytoplasmic bridges or syncytia, so once one myocyte cell membrane is activated (depolarized), a wave of excitation spreads rapidly to adjacent cells; the SA node, whose cells are relatively permeable to sodium resulting in a less negative resting potential of about –55 mV, are usually the source of spontaneous action potentials.

**Phase 0:** There is rapid opening of sodium channels with movement of sodium into the cell, the resulting electrochemical gradient leading to a positive resting membrane potential.

**Phase 1:** When membrane potential is at its most positive, the electrochemical gradient causes potassium outflow and closure of sodium channels.

**Phase 2:** A plateau phase follows, with membrane potential maintained by calcium influx; membrane potential falls towards the resting state as calcium channels gradually become inactive and potassium channels gradually open.

**Phase 3:** Potassium channels fully open, and the cell becomes repolarized.

**Phase 4:** Calcium, sodium and potassium are gradually restored to resting levels by their respective ATPase-dependent pumps.

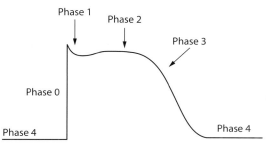

**Figure 1.2** The cardiac action potential.

Key point:    • The different phases of the cardiac action potential.

The SA node is susceptible to influence from:

- the parasympathetic nervous system via the vagus nerve, which slows heart rate
- the sympathetic nervous system via spinal nerves from T1 to T4 – these increase heart rate and can increase the force of contraction
- serum concentration of electrolytes e.g. hyperkalaemia, which can cause severe bradycardia (note that hypokalaemia can cause tachycardia)
- hypoxia, which can cause severe bradycardia.

Cardiac drugs can also affect cardiac rate, some acting through the SA node, others through the AV node or directly on ventricular myocytes:

- negative chronotropes reduce cardiac rate
  - such as beta blockers and calcium channel blockers
- positive chronotropes increase cardiac rate
  - such as dopamine and dobutamine
- negative inotropes decrease force of contraction
  - such as beta blockers, calcium channel blockers and some anti-arrhythmic drugs such as flecainide and disopyramide
- positive inotropes increase force of contraction
  - such as dopamine and dobutamine.

## THE CARDIAC CONDUCTION SYSTEM

Each normal heartbeat begins with the discharge ('depolarization') of the SA node. The impulse then spreads from the SA node to depolarise the atria. After flowing through the atria, the electrical impulse reaches the AV node, low in the right atrium.

Once the impulse has traversed the AV node, it enters the bundle of His which then divides into left and right bundle branches as it passes into the interventricular septum (Fig. 1.3). The right bundle branch conducts the wave of depolarization to the right ventricle, whereas the left bundle branch divides into anterior and posterior fascicles that conduct the wave to the left ventricle.

The conducting pathways end by dividing into Purkinje fibres that distribute the wave of depolarization rapidly throughout both ventricles. Normal depolarization of the ventricles is therefore usually very fast, occurring in less than 0.12 ms.

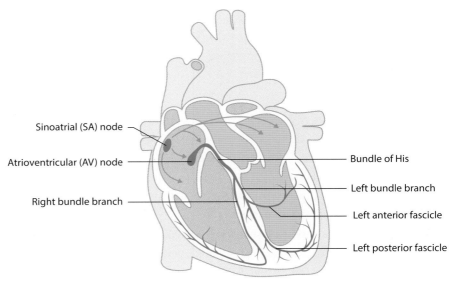

**Figure 1.3** The cardiac conduction system.

## THE CARDIAC CYCLE

The events that occur during each heartbeat are termed the cardiac cycle, commonly represented in diagrammatic form (Fig. 1.4). The cardiac cycle has four phases:

1. isovolumic contraction
2. ventricular ejection
3. isovolumic relaxation
4. ventricular filling.

These phases apply to both left and right heart, but we will focus on the left heart here for clarity. Phases 1–2 correspond with ventricular systole and phases 3–4 with ventricular diastole.

**Isovolumic contraction** begins with closure of the mitral valve, caused by the rising LV pressure at the start of ventricular systole (which coincides with the QRS complex on the ECG). After the mitral valve has closed, pressure within the LV continues to rise but the LV volume remains constant (hence 'isovolumic') until the point when the aortic valve opens.

**Ventricular ejection** commences when the aortic valve opens and blood is ejected from the LV into the aorta.

**Isovolumic relaxation** commences with closure of the aortic valve. Pressure within the LV falls during this phase (but volume remains constant), until the LV pressure falls below LA pressure. At this point, the pressure difference between LA and LV causes the mitral valve to open and isovolumic relaxation ends.

**Ventricular filling** begins as the mitral valve opens and blood flows into the LV from the LA. This phase ends when the mitral valve closes at the start of ventricular systole. Towards the end of the ventricular filling phase, atrial systole (contraction) occurs, coinciding with the P wave on the ECG, and this augments ventricular filling.

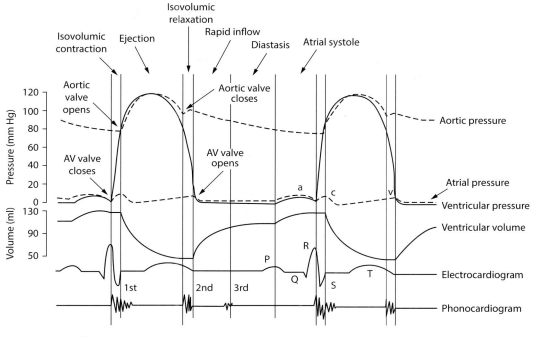

**Figure 1.4** The cardiac cycle.

Key point:  • The different phases of the cardiac cycle.

As shown in Figure 1.4, the pressures within the cardiac chambers vary through-out the cardiac cycle. A pressure difference between two chambers causes the valve between them to open or close. For example, when LA pressure exceeds LV pressure the mitral valve opens, and when LV pressure exceeds LA pressure the mitral valve closes.

## FURTHER READING

Cabrera JA, Sánchez-Quintana D. Cardiac anatomy: what the electrophysiologist needs to know. *Heart* 2013; **99**: 417–431.

Chockalingam P, Wilde A. The multifaceted cardiac sodium channel and its clinical implications. *Heart* 2012; **98**: 1318–1324.

# CHAPTER 2

# PQRST: Where the waves come from

The electrocardiogram (ECG) is one of the most widely used and useful investigations in contemporary medicine. It is essential for the identification of disorders of the cardiac rhythm, extremely useful for the diagnosis of abnormalities of the heart (such as myocardial infarction), and a helpful clue to the presence of generalized disorders that affect the rest of the body too (such as electrolyte disturbances).

Each chapter in this book considers a specific feature of the ECG in turn. We begin, however, with an overview of the ECG in which we explain the following points:

- What does the ECG actually record?
- How does the ECG 'look' at the heart?
- Where do each of the waves come from?

We recommend you take some time to read through this chapter before trying to interpret ECG abnormalities.

## WHAT DOES THE ECG ACTUALLY RECORD?

ECG machines record the electrical activity of the heart. They also pick up the activity of other muscles, such as skeletal muscle, but are designed to filter this out as much as possible. Encouraging patients to relax during an ECG recording helps to obtain a clear trace (Fig. 2.1).

By convention, the main waves on the ECG are given the names P, Q, R, S, T and U (Fig. 2.2). Each wave represents depolarization ('electrical discharging') or repolarization ('electrical recharging') of a certain region of the heart – this is discussed in more detail in the rest of this chapter.

The voltage changes detected by ECG machines are very small, being of the order of millivolts. The size of each wave corresponds to the amount of voltage

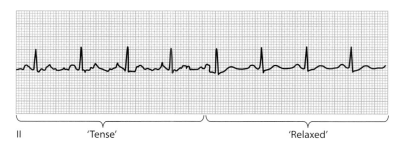

**Figure 2.1** Skeletal muscle artefact.

Key points:
- An ECG from a relaxed patient is much easier to interpret.
- Electrical interference (irregular baseline) is present when the patient is tense, but the recording is much clearer when the patient relaxes.

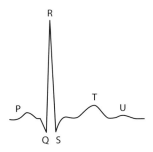

**Figure 2.2** Standard nomenclature of the ECG recording.

Key point:    • The waves are called P, Q, R, S, T and U.

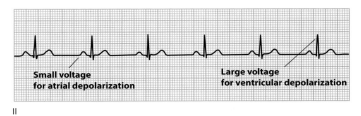

**Figure 2.3** The size of a wave reflects the voltage that caused it.

Key point:    • P waves are small (atrial depolarization generates little voltage); QRS complexes are larger (ventricular depolarization generates a higher voltage).

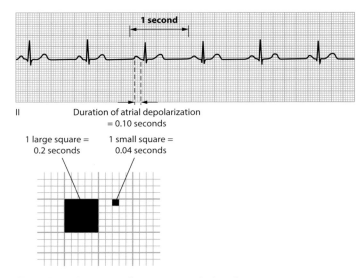

**Figure 2.4** The width of a wave reflects an event's duration.

Key points:    • The P waves are 2.5 mm wide.
     • At a paper speed of 25 mm/s, atrial depolarization therefore took 0.10 s.

generated by the event that created it: the greater the voltage, the larger the wave (Fig. 2.3).

The ECG also allows you to calculate how long an event lasted. The ECG paper moves through the machine at a constant rate of 25 mm/s, so by measuring the width of a P wave, for example, you can calculate the duration of atrial depolarization (Fig. 2.4).

# HOW DOES THE ECG 'LOOK' AT THE HEART?

To make sense of the ECG, one of the most important concepts to understand is that of the 'lead'. This is a term you will often see, and it does *not* refer to the wires that connect the patient to the ECG machine (which we will always refer to as 'electrodes' to avoid confusion).

In short, 'leads' are different *viewpoints* of the heart's electrical activity. An ECG machine uses the information it collects via its four limb and six chest electrodes to compile a comprehensive picture of the electrical activity in the heart as observed from 12 different viewpoints, and this set of 12 views or leads gives the 12-lead ECG its name.

Each lead is given a name (I, II, III, aVR, aVL, aVF, $V_1$, $V_2$, $V_3$, $V_4$, $V_5$ and $V_6$) and its position on a 12-lead ECG is usually standardized to make pattern recognition easier.

So what viewpoint does each lead have of the heart? Information from the four limb electrodes is used by the ECG machine to create the six limb leads (I, II, III, aVR, aVL and aVF). We'll say more about how the machine does this in Chapter 3. For now, you just need to know that each limb lead 'looks' at the heart from the side (the frontal or 'coronal' plane), and the view that each lead has of the heart in this plane depends on the lead in question (Fig. 2.5).

## ECG LEAD NOMENCLATURE

There are several ways of categorizing the 12 ECG leads. They are often referred to as limb leads (I, II, III, aVR, aVL, aVF) and chest leads ($V_1$, $V_2$, $V_3$, $V_4$, $V_5$, $V_6$). They can also be divided into bipolar leads (I, II, III) or unipolar leads (aVR, aVL, aVF, $V_1$, $V_2$, $V_3$, $V_4$, $V_5$, $V_6$).

Bipolar leads are generated by measuring the voltage between two electrodes – for example, lead I measures the voltage between the left arm electrode and the right arm electrode. Unipolar leads measure the voltage between a single positive electrode and a 'central' point of reference generated from the other electrodes – for example, lead aVR uses the right arm electrode as the positive pole and a combination of left arm and left leg electrodes as the negative pole.

As you can see from Figure 2.5, lead aVR looks at the heart from the approximate viewpoint of the patient's right shoulder, whereas leads I and aVL have a left lateral view of the heart, and leads II, III and aVF look at the inferior surface of the heart.

The view that each limb lead has of the heart is more formally represented in the hexaxial diagram (Fig. 2.6), which shows the angle that each limb lead has in relation to the heart. This diagram is invaluable when performing axis calculations, and we will describe how to use the diagram when we discuss the cardiac axis in Chapter 10.

The six chest leads ($V_1$–$V_6$) look at the heart in a horizontal ('transverse') plane from the front and around the side of the chest (Fig. 2.7). The region of myocardium

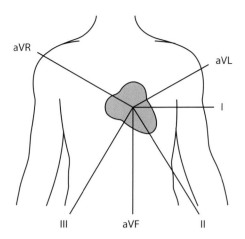

**Figure 2.5** The viewpoint each limb lead has of the heart.

Key point:   • The limb leads 'look' at the heart in the frontal (or 'coronal') plane, and each limb lead looks at the heart from a different angle.

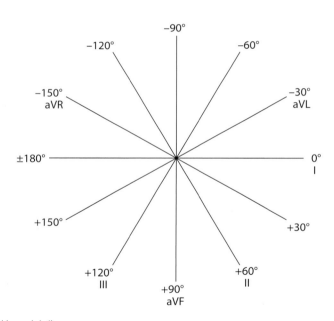

**Figure 2.6** Hexaxial diagram.

Key point:   • This shows the angle of view that each limb lead has of the heart.

surveyed by each lead therefore varies according to its vantage point – leads $V_1$–$V_4$ have an anterior view, for example, whereas leads $V_5$–$V_6$ have a lateral view.

Once you know the view each lead has of the heart, you can tell whether the electrical impulses in the heart are flowing towards that lead or away from it. This is simple to work out, because electrical current flowing towards a lead produces an upward (positive) deflection on the ECG, whereas current flowing away causes a downward (negative) deflection (Fig. 2.8).

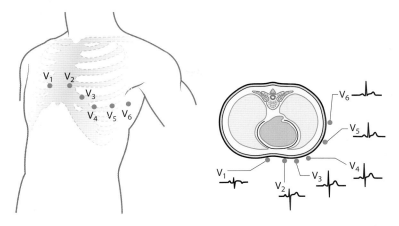

**Figure 2.7** The viewpoint each chest lead has of the heart.

Key point:   • Each chest lead looks at the heart from a different viewpoint in the horizontal ('transverse') plane.

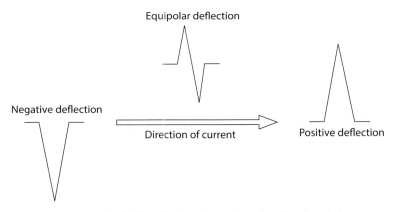

**Figure 2.8** The direction of an ECG deflection depends on the direction of the current.

Key point:   • Flow towards a lead produces a positive deflection, flow away from a lead produces a negative deflection, and flow perpendicular to a lead produces a positive then a negative (equipolar or isoelectric) deflection.

We will discuss the origin of each wave shortly, but just as an example consider the P wave, which represents atrial depolarization. The P wave is positive in lead II because atrial depolarization flows towards that lead, but it is negative in lead aVR because this lead looks at the atria from the opposite direction (Fig. 2.9).

In addition to working out the direction of flow of electrical current, knowing the viewpoint of each lead allows you to determine which regions of the heart are affected by, for example, a myocardial infarction. Infarction of the inferior surface will produce changes in the leads looking at that region, namely leads II, III and aVF (Fig. 2.10). An anterior infarction produces changes mainly in leads $V_1$–$V_4$ (Fig. 2.11).

COLOUR-CODING THE 12-LEAD ECG

As a theoretical 'concept', it has been suggested that training in ECG interpretation might be easier if 12-lead ECGs were colour-coded. The basis of the proposal is that the colours green, yellow, blue and red be printed on the 12-lead ECG paper itself to help identify the four principal 'views' of the ECG, namely:

**green** – inferior (leads II, III, aVF)
**yellow** – lateral (leads I, aVL, $V_5$–$V_6$)
**blue** – anterior ± septum (leads $V_2$–$V_4$)
**red** – right (leads aVR, $V_1$).

The colour coding could also encompass the electrodes to act as an aide-mémoire to correct placement. The right arm electrode is already coloured red (consistent with the 'right sided' view of the heart in the red-coded leads), the left arm electrode is yellow (consistent with the left lateral view in the yellow-coded leads), and the left leg electrode is green (consistent with the inferior view of the green-coded leads). With regard to the chest leads, $V_1$ could be coloured red (right of sternum), $V_2$–$V_4$ blue (left of sternum), and $V_5$–$V_6$ yellow, to match this overall scheme.

If you wish to read more about this interesting suggestion, or to see an example of a colour-coded ECG, refer to: Blakeway E, Jabbour RJ, Baksi J, Peters NS, Touquet R. ECGs: colour-coding for initial training. *Resuscitation* 2012; **83**: e115–e116 (http://dx.doi.org/10.1016/j.resuscitation.2012.01.034).

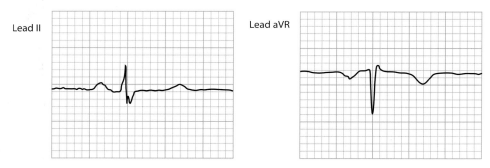

Lead II            Lead aVR

**Figure 2.9** The orientation of the P wave depends on the lead.

Key point:    • P waves are normally upright in lead II and inverted in lead aVR.

## WHERE DO EACH OF THE WAVES COME FROM?

As we saw in Chapter 1, each normal heartbeat begins with the discharge ('depolarization') of the sinoatrial (SA) node, high up in the right atrium. This is a spontaneous event, occurring 60–100 times every minute. Depolarization of the SA node does not cause any noticeable wave on the standard ECG (although it can be seen on specialized intracardiac recordings). The first detectable wave appears when the impulse spreads from the SA node to depolarize the atria (Fig. 2.12). This produces the **P wave**.

The atria contain relatively little muscle, so the voltage generated by atrial depolarization is relatively small. From the viewpoint of most leads, the electricity appears

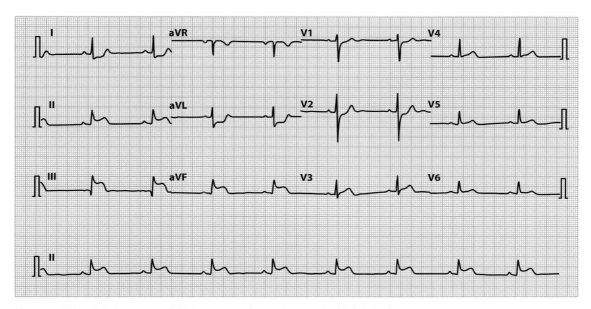

**Figure 2.10** An inferior myocardial infarction produces changes in the inferior leads.

Key points:
- Leads II, III and aVF look at the inferior surface of the heart.
- ST segment elevation is present in these leads (acute inferior myocardial infarction).
- There is also reciprocal ST segment depression in leads I and aVL.

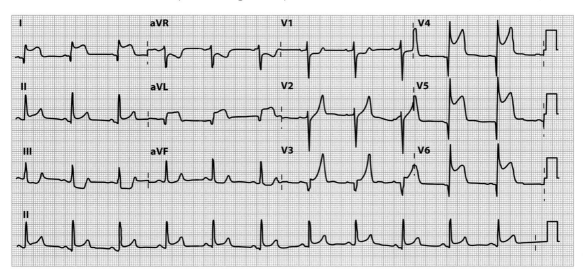

**Figure 2.11** An anterolateral myocardial infarction produces changes in the anterolateral leads.

Key points:
- Leads $V_3$–$V_6$, I and aVL look at the anterolateral surface of the heart.
- ST segment elevation is present in these leads.

to flow *towards* them and so the P wave will be a positive (upward) deflection. The exception is lead aVR, where the electricity appears to flow *away*, and so the P wave is negative in that lead (see Fig. 2.9).

After flowing through the atria, the electrical impulse reaches the atrioventricular (AV) node, low in the right atrium. Activation of the AV node does not produce

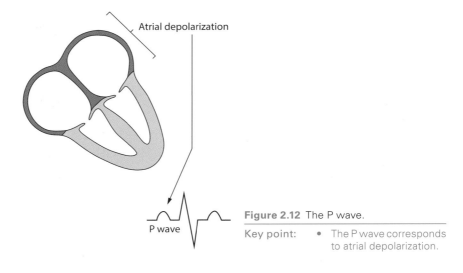

Atrial depolarization

P wave

**Figure 2.12** The P wave.

Key point:    • The P wave corresponds
                to atrial depolarization.

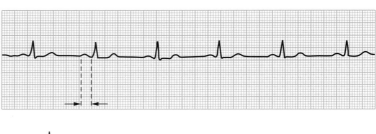

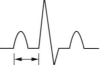

**Figure 2.13** The PR interval.

Key point:    • The PR interval is normally 0.12–0.20 s long.

an obvious wave on the ECG, but it does contribute to the time interval between the P wave and the subsequent Q or R wave. It does this by delaying conduction, and in doing so acts as a safety mechanism, preventing rapid atrial impulses (for instance during atrial flutter or fibrillation) from spreading to the ventricles at the same rate.

The time taken for the depolarization wave to pass from its origin in the SA node, across the atria, and through the AV node into ventricular muscle is called the **PR interval**. This is measured from the beginning of the P wave to the beginning of the R wave, and is normally between 0.12 s and 0.20 s, or 3 to 5 small squares on the ECG paper (Fig. 2.13).

Once the impulse has traversed the AV node, it enters the bundle of His which then divides into left and right bundle branches as it passes into the interventricular septum (Fig. 2.14). Current normally flows between the bundle branches in the interventricular septum, from left to right, and this is responsible for the

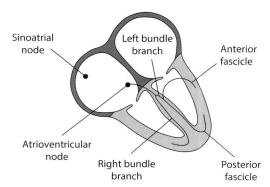

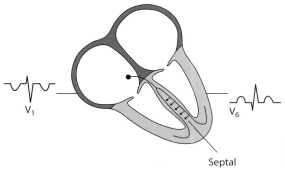

Figure 2.14 The right and left bundle branches.

Key point:    • The bundle of His divides into the right and left bundle branches in the inter.

Figure 2.15 Septal depolarization.

Key point:    • The septum normally depolarizes from left to right.

first deflection of the **QRS complex**. Whether this is a downward deflection or an upward deflection depends on which side of the septum a lead is 'looking' from (Fig. 2.15).

By convention, if the first deflection of the QRS complex is downward, it is called a **Q wave**. The first upward deflection is called an **R wave**, whether or not it follows a Q wave. A downward deflection after an R wave is called an **S wave**. Hence, a variety of complexes is possible (Fig. 2.16).

The right bundle branch conducts the wave of depolarization to the right ventricle, whereas the left bundle branch divides into anterior and posterior fascicles that conduct the wave to the left ventricle (Fig. 2.17). The conducting pathways end by dividing into Purkinje fibres that distribute the wave of depolarization rapidly throughout both ventricles. The depolarization of the ventricles, represented by the QRS complex, is normally complete within 0.12 s (Fig. 2.18). QRS complexes are 'positive' or 'negative', depending on whether the R wave or the S wave is bigger (Fig. 2.19). This, in turn, will depend on the view each lead has of the heart.

The left ventricle contains considerably more myocardium than the right, and so the voltage generated by its depolarization will tend to dominate the shape of the QRS complex.

Leads that look at the heart from the right will see a relatively small amount of voltage moving towards them as the right ventricle depolarizes, and a larger amount moving away with depolarization of the left ventricle. The QRS complex will therefore be dominated by an S wave, and be negative. Conversely, leads

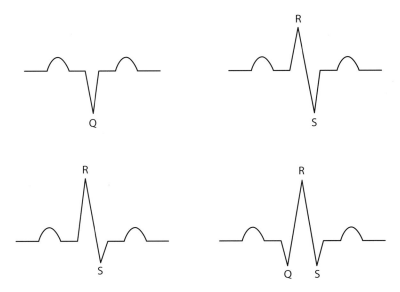

**Figure 2.16** The different varieties of QRS complex.

Key point:   • The first downward deflection is a Q wave, the first upward deflection is an R wave, and a downward deflection after an R wave is an S wave.

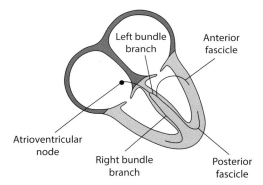

**Figure 2.17** Divisions of the left bundle branch.

Key point:   • The left bundle branch divides into anterior and posterior fascicles.

looking at the heart from the left will see a relatively large voltage moving towards them, and a smaller voltage moving away, giving rise to a large R wave and only a small S wave (Fig. 2.20). Therefore, there is a gradual transition across the chest leads, from a predominantly negative QRS complex to a predominantly positive one (Fig. 2.21).

The **ST segment** is the transient period in which no more electrical current can be passed through the myocardium. It is measured from the end of the S wave to the beginning of the T wave (Fig. 2.22). The ST segment is of particular interest in the diagnosis of myocardial infarction and ischaemia (see Chapter 15).

The **T wave** represents repolarization ('recharging') of the ventricular myocardium to its resting electrical state. The **QT interval** measures the total time for activation of the ventricles and recovery to the normal resting state (Fig. 2.23).

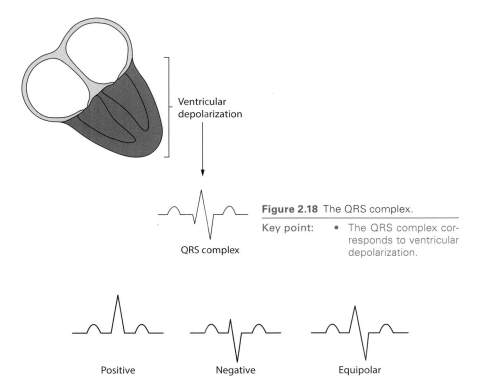

**Figure 2.18** The QRS complex.

Key point: • The QRS complex corresponds to ventricular depolarization.

**Figure 2.19** Polarity of the QRS complexes.

Key point: • A dominant R wave means a positive QRS complex, a dominant S wave means a negative QRS complex, and equal R and S waves mean an equipolar (isoelectric) QRS complex.

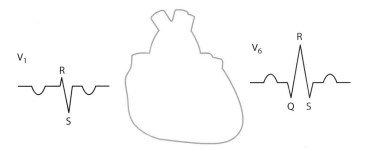

**Figure 2.20** The shape of the QRS complex depends on the lead's viewpoint.

Key point: • Right-sided leads have negative QRS complexes, and left-sided leads have positive QRS complexes.

The origin of the **U wave** is uncertain, but it may represent repolarization of the interventricular septum or slow repolarization of the ventricles. U waves can be difficult to identify but, when present, they are most clearly seen in the anterior chest leads $V_2$–$V_3$ (Fig. 18.2).

You need to be familiar with the most important electrical events that make up the cardiac cycle. These are summarized at the end of the chapter.

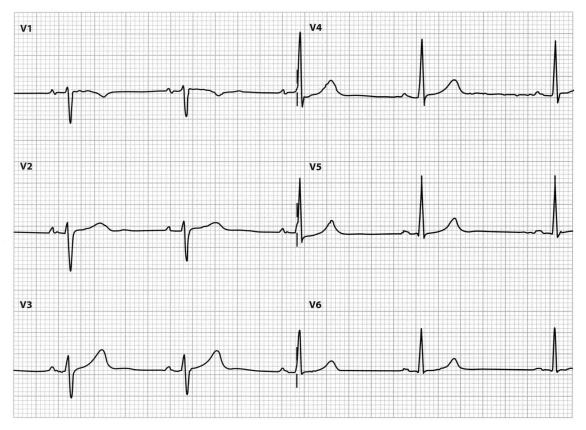

**Figure 2.21** Transition in QRS complexes across the chest leads.

Key point:    • QRS complexes are normally negative in leads $V_1$ and $V_2$ and positive in leads $V_5$ and $V_6$.

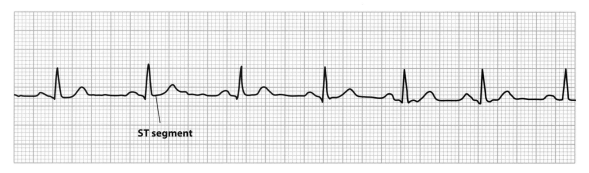

**Figure 2.22** The ST segment.

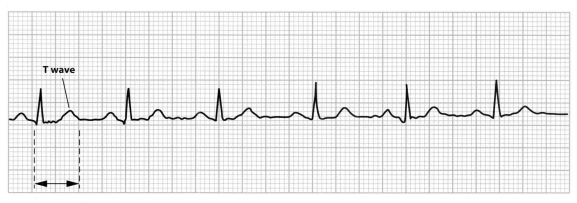

0.39 seconds

**Figure 2.23** The T wave and QT interval.

## SUMMARY

The waves and intervals of the ECG correspond to the following events:

| ECG event | Cardiac event |
| --- | --- |
| P wave | Atrial depolarization |
| PR interval | Start of atrial depolarization to start of ventricular depolarization |
| QRS complex | Ventricular depolarization |
| ST segment | Pause in ventricular electrical activity before repolarization |
| T wave | Ventricular repolarization |
| QT interval | Total time taken by ventricular depolarization and repolarization |
| U wave | Uncertain – possibly:<br>• interventricular septal repolarization<br>• slow ventricular repolarization |

*Note:* Depolarizations of the SA and AV nodes are important events but do not in themselves produce a detectable wave on the standard ECG.

## FURTHER READING

Blakeway E, Jabbour RJ, Baksi J, *et al.* ECGs: colour-coding for initial training. *Resuscitation* 2012; **83**: e115–e116.

Hurst JW. Naming of the waves in the ECG, with a brief account of their genesis. *Circulation* 1998; **98**: 1937–1942.

# CHAPTER 3

# Performing an ECG recording

This guide to performing a standard 12-lead ECG recording is based upon the current clinical guidelines of the Society for Cardiological Science and Technology in the United Kingdom (see *Further Reading*). Anyone performing a 12-lead ECG recording should have received appropriate training and been assessed in their skills by a competent practitioner.

## INITIAL PREPARATIONS

Before making a 12-lead ECG recording, check that the ECG machine is safe to use and has been cleaned appropriately. Before you start, ensure you have an adequate supply of:

- recording paper
- skin preparation equipment
- electrodes.

Introduce yourself to the patient and confirm their identity. Explain what you plan to do and why, and ensure that they consent to undergo the ECG recording.

The 12-lead ECG should be recorded with the patient in a recumbent position on a couch or bed, in a warm environment, while ensuring that the patient is comfortable and able to relax. This is not only important for patient dignity, but also helps to ensure a high-quality recording with minimal artefact.

### Skin preparation

In order to apply the electrodes, the patient's skin needs to be exposed across the chest, the arms and the lower legs. Ensure that you follow your local chaperone policy, and offer the patient a gown to cover any exposed areas once the electrodes are applied.

To optimize electrode contact with the patient's skin and reduce 'noise', consider the following tips:

- removal of chest hair
  - It may be necessary to remove chest hair in the areas where the electrodes are to be applied. Ensure the patient consents to this before you start. Carry a supply of disposable razors on your ECG cart for this purpose.
- light abrasion
  - Exfoliation of the skin using light abrasion can help improve electrode contact. This can be achieved using specially manufactured abrasive tape or by using a paper towel.
- skin cleansing
  - An alcohol wipe helps to remove grease from the surface of the skin, although this may be better avoided if patients have fragile or broken skin.

- electrode placement
    - Correct placement of ECG electrodes is essential to ensure that the 12-lead ECG can be interpreted correctly. Electrode misplacement is a common occurrence, reported in 0.4% of ECGs recorded in the cardiac outpatient clinic and 4.0% of ECGs recorded in the Intensive Care Unit.

The standard 12-lead ECG consists of:

- three bipolar limb leads (I, II and III)
- three augmented limb leads (aVR, aVL and aVF)
- six chest (or 'precordial') leads ($V_1$–$V_6$).

As we saw in Chapter 2, these 12 leads are generated using 10 ECG electrodes, four of which are applied to the limbs and six of which are applied to the chest. The ECG electrodes are colour coded; however, two different colour coding systems exist internationally. In Europe, the IEC (International Electrotechnical Commission) system uses the following colour codes:

| | |
|---|---|
| Right arm | Red |
| Left arm | Yellow |
| Right leg | Black |
| Left leg | Green |
| Chest $V_1$ | White/red |
| Chest $V_2$ | White/yellow |
| Chest $V_3$ | White/green |
| Chest $V_4$ | White/brown |
| Chest $V_5$ | White/black |
| Chest $V_6$ | White/violet |

To help you in placing the limb electrodes, remember the mnemonic 'Ride Your Green Bike'. Start by attaching the red ('Ride') electrode on the patient's right arm, then move around the patient's torso clockwise, attaching the yellow ('Your') electrode on the left arm, then the green ('Green') electrode on the left leg, and finally the black ('Bike') electrode on the right leg.

In the United States the AHA (American Heart Association) system uses a different set of colour codes:

| | |
|---|---|
| Right arm | White |
| Left arm | Black |
| Right leg | Green |
| Left leg | Red |
| Chest $V_1$ | Brown/red |
| Chest $V_2$ | Brown/yellow |
| Chest $V_3$ | Brown/green |
| Chest $V_4$ | Brown/blue |
| Chest $V_5$ | Brown/orange |
| Chest $V_6$ | Brown/purple |

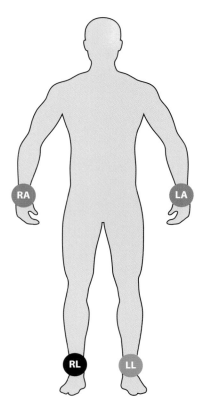

**Figure 3.1** Placement of the limb electrodes.

Key point:    • The electrodes are placed on the right arm (RA), left arm (LA), right leg (RL) and left leg (LL).

## PLACEMENT OF THE LIMB ELECTRODES

The four limb electrodes should be attached to the arms and legs just proximal to the wrist and ankle (Fig. 3.1). If the electrodes have to be placed in a more proximal position on the limb (perhaps because of leg ulcers or a previous amputation), this should be noted on the ECG recording. Placing the limb electrodes more proximally on the limbs can alter the appearance of the ECG and it is therefore important that the person interpreting the recording is aware that an atypical electrode position has been used.

## PLACEMENT OF THE CHEST (PRECORDIAL) ELECTRODES

The six chest electrodes should be positioned on the chest wall as shown in Figure 3.2. Common errors, which should be avoided, include placing electrodes $V_1$ and $V_2$ too high and $V_5$ and $V_6$ too low. The correct location is:

| | |
|---|---|
| Chest $V_1$ | 4th intercostal space, right sternal edge |
| Chest $V_2$ | 4th intercostal space, left sternal edge |
| Chest $V_3$ | Midway in between $V_2$ and $V_4$ |
| Chest $V_4$ | 5th intercostal space, mid-clavicular line |
| Chest $V_5$ | Left anterior axillary line, same horizontal level as $V_4$ |
| Chest $V_6$ | Left mid-axillary line, same horizontal level as $V_4$ and $V_5$ |

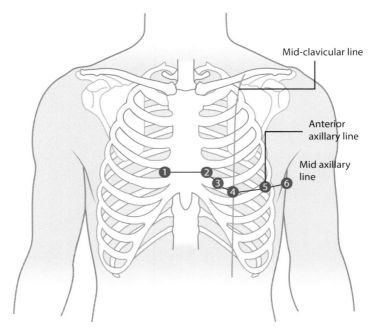

**Figure 3.2** Placement of the chest (precordial) electrodes.

As with the limb electrodes, any variation from the standard locations should be noted on the ECG recording to avoid misinterpretation.

The simplest way to count the rib spaces is to begin by finding the angle of Louis, the horizontal bony ridge part way down the sternum. Run a finger down from the top of the sternum until you feel this ridge, and then run your finger sideways and slightly downwards to the patient's right until you reach a space between the ribs and the right-hand edge of the sternum – this is the 2nd intercostal space. Count down the rib spaces with your fingers to the 3rd and then the 4th intercostal space, and this is where you place electrode $V_1$. The equivalent space at the left sternal edge is the location for electrode $V_2$.

Next, staying to the left of the sternum count down to the 5th intercostal space and find the mid-clavicular line – this is the location for electrode $V_4$. Electrode $V_3$ can then be positioned midway between $V_2$ and $V_4$.

Then, move horizontally from electrode $V_4$ to the patient's left until you reach the anterior axillary line. This is the location for electrode $V_5$. It is important to ensure that you do not follow the rib space round to $V_5$, but stay horizontal. Finally, remaining in a horizontal line with $V_4$, place electrode $V_6$ in the mid-axillary line.

FEMALE PATIENTS

Placement of the chest electrodes can sometimes pose difficulties in female patients because of the left breast. By convention, the electrodes $V_4$–$V_6$ are placed *underneath* the left breast.

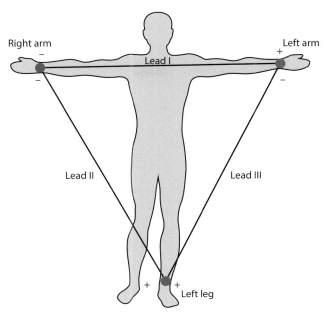

**Figure 3.3** Einthoven's triangle, formed by the placement of the right arm (RA), left arm (LA) and left leg (LL) electrodes.

## EINTHOVEN'S TRIANGLE

Before we record the ECG, it is worth pausing for a moment to consider how the electrodes we have attached actually make the recording. If we consider the three bipolar limb leads I, II and III to begin with, these are generated by the ECG machine using various pairings of the left arm (LA), right arm (RA) and left leg (LL) electrodes (Fig. 3.3). The three limb leads are called 'bipolar' leads because they are generated from the potential difference between pairs of these limb electrodes:

- lead I is recorded using RA as the negative pole, and LA as the positive pole
- lead II is recorded using RA as the negative pole, and LL as the positive pole
- lead III is recorded using LA as the negative pole, and LL as the positive pole.

If you measure the potential differences in each of these three limb leads at any one moment, they are linked by the equation:

$$II = I + III$$

In other words, the net voltage in lead II will always equal the sum of the net voltages in leads I and III. This is known as **Einthoven's Law**. You can see this in action in Figure 3.4. In this ECG:

- the R wave in lead I measures 5 mm, with no significant S wave, giving a net size of 5 mm (or 0.5 mV)
- the R wave in lead III measures 3.5 mm, with an S wave of 2.5 mm, giving a net size of 1 mm (or 0.1 mV).

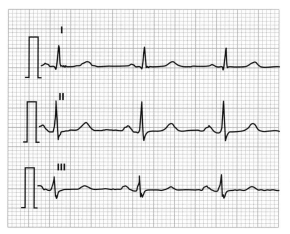

**Figure 3.4** Leads I, II and III.

Key point:
- According to Einthoven's Law, the net voltage in lead II will always equal the sum of the net voltages in leads I and III.

Using Einthoven's Law:

$$II = I + III$$

$$II = 0.5 \text{ mV} + 0.1 \text{ mV}$$

$$II = 0.6 \text{ mV}$$

If you look at lead II in Figure 3.4, there is an R wave of 8 mm and an S wave of 2 mm, so the net size of the QRS complex is, as we predicted, 6 mm (or 0.6 mV).

**Einthoven's triangle**, as represented in Figure 3.3, can be simplified and represented as in Figure 3.5. This can be further represented as in Figure 3.6, with the vectors all centred on the same point, which makes it clearer as to how leads I, II and III achieve their 'view' of the heart. Compare this to the hexaxial diagram in Figure 2.6, and it should now be a little easier to visualize how the limb electrodes RA, LA and LL relate to the leads I, II and III, and how these leads' views of the heart come about.

What about the other three limb leads, aVR, aVL and aVF? These leads are generated in a similar way to leads I, II and III. However, this time *two* of the electrodes are *combined* to form the negative pole, and the other electrode acts as the positive pole. Hence:

- lead aVR is recorded using LA+LL as the negative pole, and RA as the positive pole
- lead aVL is recorded using RA+LL as the negative pole, and LA as the positive pole
- lead aVF is recorded using RA+LA as the negative pole, and LL as the positive pole.

Figure 3.7 shows how these three leads can be represented diagrammatically, with regard to their vectors and therefore their views of the heart. Again, this corresponds to the angles shown in the hexaxial diagram in Figure 2.6.

What about the chest leads, $V_1$–$V_6$? For these leads, the negative pole is generated by combining the electrodes RA, LA and LL together. This combination of all three limb electrodes – which is known as **Wilson's central terminal** – gives the

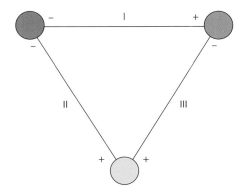

**Figure 3.5** Einthoven's triangle, simplified as an equilateral triangle.

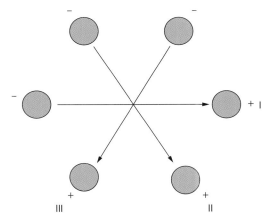

**Figure 3.6** Einthoven's triangle, with all three vectors centred on the same point.

average potential across the body, which approximates to zero. Each of the six chest leads uses the relevant chest electrode as a positive pole to measure the potential difference.

A more detailed yet very clear discussion of Einthoven's triangle can be found online at: http://ems12lead.com/tag/einthovens-triangle/.

---

### THE RIGHT LEG ELECTRODE

You may have noticed that the right leg electrode (RL) hasn't featured so far in the discussion about how the ECG leads are generated. So what does the RL electrode actually do? RL is used by the ECG machine as a 'reference' electrode to help reduce unwanted 'noise' during the recording.

---

## RECORDING THE 12-LEAD ECG

Ensure that the patient's name and other relevant identification details (e.g. date of birth, hospital number) have been entered into the ECG, and that the machine

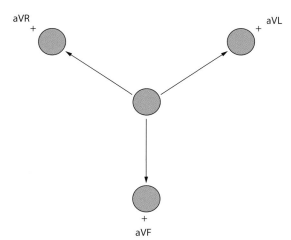

**Figure 3.7** Leads aVR, aVL and aVF, represented diagrammatically.

is displaying the correct date and time. Encourage the patient to relax while the recording is being made, and check that the patient is lying still and not clenching their muscles.

Do not use a filter for the initial recording; however, if necessary the recording can be repeated with the filter switched on if the initial recording shows 'noise'.

### ECG MACHINE FILTERS

ECG machines offer a number of types of filter to try and improve the quality of the ECG signal. A low-frequency filter (also known as a high-pass filter) is used to filter out low-frequency signals, typically anything less than 0.05 Hz, to reduce baseline drift. A high-frequency (or low-pass) filter is used to filter out high-frequency signals, typically anything over 100 Hz, to reduce interference from skeletal muscle. A 'notch' filter is specifically designed to filter out noise at a specific frequency and can be used to reduce electrical alternating current 'hum' at 50 or 60 Hz. While filtering can improve the appearance of the ECG, it can also introduce distortion, particularly of the ST segments, and thus should only be used when necessary. For this reason, ECGs should always initially be recorded with the filters off, and repeated with the filters on only if needed.

Make the ECG recording at a paper speed of 25 mm/s and a gain setting of 10 mm/mV. If however the ECG contains high-voltage complexes (as in left ventricular hypertrophy, p. 146), repeat the recording at a gain setting of 5 mm/mV (ensuring that this is clearly marked on the ECG).

Once the recording has been made, check that it is of good quality and ensure that all the patient details are correctly shown on it. If the patient was experiencing any symptoms at the time of the recording (such as chest pain or palpitations), note this on the recording as such information can prove very useful diagnostically. If the patient was experiencing symptoms during the recording, or if the recording shows any clinically urgent abnormalities, report this information to a more senior staff member as appropriate.

Once you are satisfied with the ECG recording, detach the electrodes from the patient and assist them in getting dressed. Ensure that the materials used during the recording are disposed of safely and appropriately.

---

**ECG RECORDINGS IN DEXTROCARDIA**

In dextrocardia, the heart is located on the right side of the chest rather than on the left (p. 149). Dextrocardia is suggested by poor R wave progression across the chest leads and by P wave inversion in lead I. If a patient has known or suspected dextrocardia, repeat the recording with the chest electrodes positioned in a mirror image on the right side of the chest. Ensure the ECG is labelled clearly with $V_3R$, $V_4R$ etc. to demonstrate that right-sided chest electrodes have been used. The limb electrodes are usually left in their standard positions, as this helps to 'flag up' the apparent dextrocardia on the ECG, but if you do prefer to reverse the limb electrodes too then it is essential to label the reversed limb leads clearly on the ECG. Ensure that copies of *both* ECGs (the standard one and the one with right-sided electrodes) are retained.

---

## SUMMARY

To record an optimal 12-lead ECG:

- explain the procedure to the patient and obtain their consent
- ensure the patient is comfortable
- prepare the skin before applying the electrodes
    - removal of chest hair
    - light abrasion
    - skin cleansing
- place the electrodes correctly
- only use ECG filters where necessary, and note this on the ECG
- check that the ECG recording is of good quality
- label the ECG recording appropriately
- ensure that any clinically urgent abnormalities are acted upon.

## FURTHER READING

Kligfield P, Gettes LS, Bailey JJ, *et al*. AHA/ACCF/HRS recommendations for the standardization and interpretation of the electrocardiogram: Part I: The electrocardiogram and its technology. *J Am Coll Cardiol* 2007; **49**: 1109–1127.

Macfarlane PW, Coleman EN. Resting 12 lead ECG electrode placement and associated problems. 1995. Published by The Society for Cardiological Science and Technology. Available for download from www.scst.org.uk.

Rudiger A, Hellermann JP, Mukherjee R, *et al*. Electrocardiographic artifacts due to electrode misplacement and their frequency in different clinical settings. *Am J Emerg Med* 2007; **25**: 174–178.

The Society for Cardiological Science and Technology: Clinical Guidelines by Consensus. Recording a standard 12-lead electrocardiogram: an approved methodology. February 2010. Available for download from www.scst.org.uk.

# CHAPTER 4

# Reporting an ECG recording

The reporting of an ECG recording is best done in a methodical manner to ensure that your report is comprehensive and doesn't overlook any potentially important details. In this chapter we will give you a systematic overview of how to approach a 12-lead ECG, and all of these points will be expanded upon in the chapters that follow.

Your everyday reports may not need to be as detailed as the one presented at the end of this chapter, but it is nonetheless good practice to have a thorough 'mental checklist' to work through as your review an ECG to ensure that all the key findings are covered.

## PATIENT DATA

Begin by checking key information on the ECG and/or request form relating to the patient:

- patient name
- date of birth
- identification number (e.g. hospital number)
- reason for the request
- relevant past medical history
- relevant medication.

## TECHNICAL DATA

Next, report on technical data pertaining to the recording, namely:

- date and time of recording
- paper speed and calibration
- technical quality
- any atypical settings
- additional leads (e.g. posterior leads, right-sided chest leads)
- physiological manoeuvres (e.g. ECG recorded during deep inspiration)
- diagnostic or therapeutic manoeuvres (e.g. ECG recorded during carotid sinus massage).

## ECG FUNDAMENTALS

Next, report on the fundamental features of the ECG recording itself, namely:

- rate
- rhythm
  - supraventricular

- ventricular
- conduction problems
- axis.

## ECG DETAILS

Next, review the individual features of the ECG using a step-by-step approach. Describe:

- P wave
- PR interval
- Q wave
- QRS complex
- ST segment
- T wave
- QT interval
- U wave.

Don't overlook any additional features, such as:

- delta wave
- J wave (Osborn wave).

## REPORT SUMMARY

Finally, end your report with a summary of the key ECG findings, placing them where possible in the context of the clinical information provided.

---

*This 12-lead ECG was performed on Mr John Smith, born on 1 January 1950, hospital number 123456. The request form states that the patient is experiencing breathlessness and irregular palpitations. He has a history of inferior myocardial infarction in 2011. He is currently taking aspirin, simvastatin, bisoprolol and ramipril.*

*The recording was performed on 1 August 2013, using a paper speed of 25 mm/s and a calibration of 10 mm/mV. The recording is of good quality with no artefact.*

*The ventricular rate is tachycardic at 114/min. The rhythm is atrial fibrillation, as evidence by no co-ordinated atrial activity and irregularly irregular QRS complexes. The QRS axis is normal at +64°.*

*The P waves are absent and so the PR interval cannot be measured. There are deep Q waves and inverted T waves in the inferior leads. The remainder of the QRS complexes are unremarkable. The ST segments are normal. The QT interval is normal (QTc measures 428 ms). There are no U waves present.*

***In conclusion,*** *this 12-lead ECG shows:*

- *atrial fibrillation with a fast ventricular rate (114/min)*
- *inferior Q waves and T wave inversion, consistent with an old inferior myocardial infarction.*

Your complete report may read like this:

If you have old ECGs for comparison, you may wish to include details of any relevant changes in the ECG in your report (e.g. new evidence of myocardial infarction, new conduction problems, changes in rhythm etc.).

---

## SUMMARY

To report a 12-lead ECG, review the following features:

- patient data
  - patient name
  - date of birth
  - identification number (e.g. hospital number)
  - reason for the request
  - relevant past medical history
  - relevant medication
- technical data
  - date and time of recording
  - paper speed and calibration
  - technical quality
  - any non-standard settings
- ECG fundamentals
  - rate
  - rhythm
  - axis
- ECG details
  - P wave
  - PR interval
  - Q wave
  - QRS complex
  - ST segment
  - T wave
  - QT interval
  - U wave
  - additional features (delta wave, J wave)

Conclude your ECG report with a summary of the key findings.

## FURTHER READING

Mason JW, Hancock EW, Gettes LS. AHA/ACCF/HRS recommendations for the standardization and interpretation of the electrocardiogram: Part II: Electrocardiography diagnostic statement list. *J Am Coll Cardiol* 2007; **49**: 1128–1135.

Measurement of the heart rate and the identification of the cardiac rhythm go hand in hand, as many abnormalities of heart rate result from arrhythmias. The following chapters discuss in detail how to identify the cardiac rhythm. To begin with, however, we will simply describe ways to measure the heart rate and the abnormalities that can affect it.

When we talk of measuring the heart rate, we usually mean the *ventricular* rate, which corresponds to the patient's pulse. Depolarization of the ventricles produces the QRS complex on the ECG, and so it is the rate of QRS complexes that needs to be measured to determine the heart rate.

Measurement of the heart rate is simple and can be done in several ways. However, before you try to measure anything, check that the ECG has been recorded at the standard UK and US paper speed of 25 mm/s. If so, then all you have to remember is that a 1-min ECG tracing covers **300 large squares**. If the patient's rhythm is regular, all you have to do is count the number of large squares between two consecutive QRS complexes, and divide it into 300.

For example, in Figure 5.1 there are approximately 4 large squares between each QRS complex. Therefore:

$$\text{Heart rate} = \frac{300}{4} = 75 \, / \min$$

An alternative, and slightly more accurate, method is to count small squares rather than big ones. For this method, you need to remember than a 1-min ECG tracing covers **1500 small squares**. Count the number of small squares between two consecutive QRS complexes, and divide it into 1500.

Using the ECG in Figure 5.1, there are 21 small squares between each QRS complex. Therefore:

$$\text{Heart rate} = \frac{1500}{21} = 71 \, / \min$$

This method does not work so well when the rhythm is irregular, as the number of large squares between each QRS complex varies from beat to beat. So, instead, count the number of QRS complexes in 50 large squares (Fig. 5.2) – the length of the rhythm strip on a standard ECG. This is the number of QRS complexes in 10 s. To work out the rate/min, simply multiply by 6:

Number of QRS complexes in 50 large squares = 19

Therefore, number of QRS complexes in 10 s = 19

Therefore, number of QRS complexes/min = 19 × 6 = 114

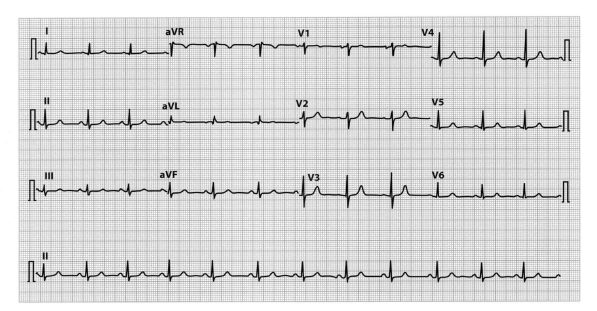

**Figure 5.1** Calculating heart rate when the rhythm is regular.

Key points:
- There are approximately 4 large squares between each QRS complex, corresponding to a heart rate of approximately 75/min.
- More precisely, there are 21 small squares between each QRS complex, giving a more accurate heart rate of 71/min.

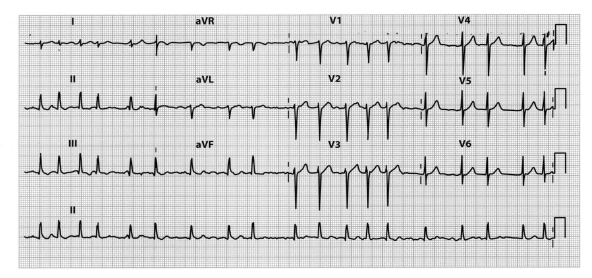

**Figure 5.2** Calculating heart rate when the rhythm is irregular.

Key point:
- There are 19 QRS complexes in 50 large squares (10 s), corresponding to a heart rate of 114/min.

An ECG ruler can be helpful, but follow the instructions on it carefully. Some ECG machines will calculate heart rate and print it on the ECG, but always check machine-derived values, as the machines do occasionally make errors!

Whichever method you use, remember it can also be used to measure the atrial or P wave rate as well as the ventricular or QRS rate. Normally, every P wave is followed

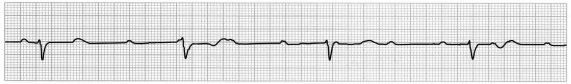

Lead II

**Figure 5.3** The P wave rate can differ from the QRS complex rate.

Key point:    • This rhythm strip shows third-degree AV block, with a P wave (atrial) rate of 94/min and a QRS complex (ventricular) rate of 33/min.

by a QRS complex and so the atrial and ventricular rates are the same. However, the rates can be different if, for example, some or all of the P waves are prevented from activating the ventricles (Fig. 5.3). Situations where this may happen are described in later chapters.

Once you have measured the heart rate, you need to decide whether it is normal or abnormal. As a general rule, a regular heart rhythm with a rate between 60 and 100/min is normal. If the rate is below 60/min, the patient is said to be **bradycardic**. With a heart rate above 100/min, the patient is **tachycardic**. Therefore, the two questions you need to ask about heart rate are:

● Is the heart rate below 60/min?

● Is the heart rate above 100/min?

If the answer to either question is 'yes', turn to the appropriate half of this chapter to find out what to do next. If not, turn to Chapter 6 to start your identification of the cardiac rhythm.

## IS THE HEART RATE BELOW 60/MIN?

**Bradycardia** is arbitrarily defined as a heart rate below 60/min. Identification of the cardiac rhythm and any conduction disturbances is essential, and this is discussed in the following chapters.

Problems to consider in the bradycardic patient are:

● sinus bradycardia

● sick sinus syndrome

● second-degree and third-degree atrioventricular (AV) block

● 'escape' rhythms

● AV junctional escape rhythm

● ventricular escape rhythms

● asystole.

**Sinus bradycardia** (p. 54) can be normal, for example in athletes during sleep, but in others it may indicate an underlying problem. The differential diagnosis and treatment are discussed in Chapter 7.

**Table 5.1** Common negatively chronotropic drugs

- Beta blockers (do not forget eye drops)
- Some calcium antagonists, e.g. verapamil, diltiazem
- Digoxin
- Ivabradine

**Sick sinus syndrome** (p. 57) is the coexistence of sinus bradycardia with episodes of sinus arrest and sinoatrial block. Patients may also have episodes of paroxysmal tachycardia, giving rise to the tachy-brady syndrome.

In **second-degree AV block** (p. 94) some atrial impulses fail to be conducted to the ventricles, and this can lead to bradycardia. In **third-degree AV block**, no atrial impulses can reach the ventricles; in response, the ventricles usually develop an 'escape' rhythm (see below). It is important to remember that AV block can coexist with *any* atrial rhythm.

**Escape rhythms** are a form of 'safety net' to maintain a heart beat if the normal mechanism of impulse generation fails or is blocked. They may also appear during episodes of severe sinus bradycardia. Escape rhythms are discussed in more detail in Chapter 9 (p. 102).

**Asystole** (p. 47) implies the absence of ventricular activity, and so the heart rate is zero. Asystole is a medical emergency and requires immediate diagnosis and treatment if the patient is to have any chance of survival.

Do not forget that arrhythmias that are usually associated with normal or fast heart rates may be slowed by certain drugs, resulting in bradycardia. For example, patients with atrial fibrillation (which if untreated may cause a *tachycardia*) can develop a bradycardia when commenced on anti-arrhythmic drugs. Table 5.1 lists drugs that commonly slow the heart rate (**negatively chronotropic**). A thorough review of all the patient's current and recent medications is therefore essential.

**DRUG POINT**

A complete drug history is essential in any patient with an abnormal ECG.

The first step in managing a bradycardia is to assess the urgency of the situation – in the peri-arrest situation, use the ABCDE approach and assess the patient for adverse features (p. 39). The Resuscitation Council (UK) 2010 algorithm on the immediate management of bradycardia in adults is shown in Figure 5.4. The longer-term management of specific bradycardias is discussed in the chapters which follow.

## IS THE HEART RATE ABOVE 100/MIN?

**Tachycardia** is arbitrarily defined as a heart rate above 100/min. When a patient presents with a tachycardia, begin by identifying the cardiac rhythm. See Chapter 6

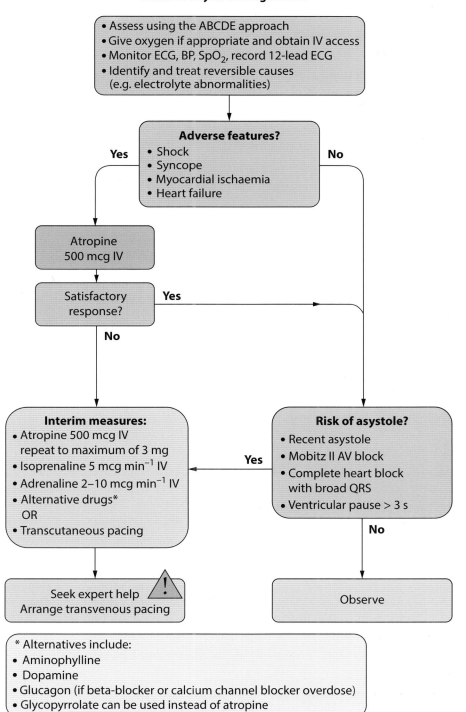

**Figure 5.4** Resuscitation Council (UK) 2010 adult bradycardia algorithm. Reproduced with the kind permission of the Resuscitation Council (UK).

for an approach to recognizing cardiac rhythms. Begin the process of identification by checking whether the QRS complexes are:

- narrow (<3 small squares)
- broad (>3 small squares).

**Narrow-complex tachycardias** always arise from above the ventricles – that is, they are supraventricular in origin. The possibilities are:

- sinus tachycardia
- atrial tachycardia
- atrial flutter
- atrial fibrillation
- AV re-entry tachycardia (AVRT)
- AV nodal re-entry tachycardia (AVNRT).

All of these are discussed in detail in Chapter 7.

Broad QRS complexes can occur if normal electrical impulses are conducted abnormally or 'aberrantly' to the ventricles. This delays ventricular activation, widening the QRS complex. Any of the supraventricular tachycardias (SVTs) listed above can also present as a **broad-complex tachycardia** if aberrant conduction is present.

Broad-complex tachycardia should also make you think of ventricular arrhythmias:

- ventricular tachycardia
- accelerated idioventricular rhythm
- torsades de pointes.

Each of these, including aberrant conduction, is discussed in Chapter 8. How to distinguish between ventricular tachycardia and SVT with aberrant conduction is discussed on page 86.

Ventricular fibrillation (VF, p. 90) is hard to categorize. The chaotic nature of the underlying ventricular activity can give rise to a variety of ECG appearances, but all have the characteristics of being unpredictable and chaotic. Ventricular fibrillation is a medical emergency and so it is important that you can recognize it immediately.

Management of tachycardia depends on the underlying rhythm, and the treatment of the different arrhythmias is detailed in the following chapters. The first step, as with managing a bradycardia, is to assess the urgency of the situation – in the peri-arrest situation, use the ABCDE approach and assess the patient for adverse features (p. 39). The Resuscitation Council (UK) 2010 algorithm on the immediate management of tachycardia (with a pulse) in adults is shown in Figure 5.5. The longer-term management of specific tachycardias is discussed in the chapters which follow.

Clues to the nature of the arrhythmia may be found in the patient's history. Ask the patient about:

- how any palpitations start and stop (sudden or gradual)
- whether there are any situations in which they are more likely to happen (e.g. during exercise, lying quietly in bed)

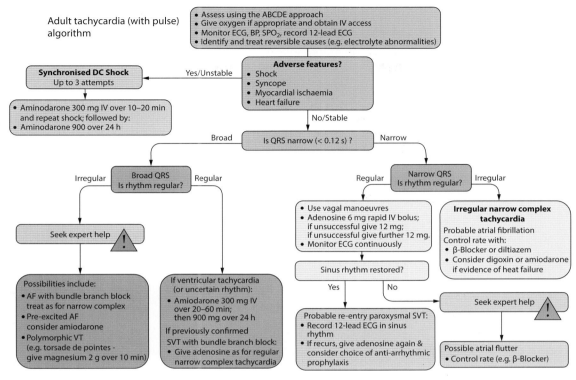

**Figure 5.5** Resuscitation Council (UK) 2010 adult tachycardia (with a pulse) algorithm. AF – atrial fibrillation; SVT – supraventricular tachycardia; VT – ventricular tachycardia. Reproduced with the kind permission of the Resuscitation Council (UK).

- how long they last
- whether there are any associated symptoms (dizziness, syncope, falls, fatigue, breathlessness and chest pain).

Also ask the patient to 'tap out' how the palpitations feel – this will give you clues about the rate (fast or slow) and rhythm (regular or irregular).

Also enquire about symptoms of related disorders (e.g. hyperthyroidism) and obtain a list of current medications. Check for any drugs (e.g. salbutamol) that can increase the heart rate (**positively chronotropic**). Do not forget to ask about caffeine intake (coffee, tea and cola drinks).

A thorough examination is always important, looking for evidence of haemodynamic disturbance (hypotension, cardiac failure and poor peripheral perfusion) and coexistent disorders (e.g. thyroid goitre).

Use the history, examination and further investigations (e.g. plasma electrolytes, thyroid function tests) to reach a diagnosis. Ambulatory ECG recording may be helpful if circumstances permit it (see Chapter 21).

## SUMMARY

To assess the heart rate, ask the following questions.

*1. Is the heart rate below 60/min?*

If 'yes', consider:

- sinus bradycardia
- sick sinus syndrome
- second-degree and third-degree AV block
- escape rhythms
    - AV junctional escape rhythm
    - ventricular escape rhythms
- asystole.

*2. Is the heart rate above 100/min?*

If 'yes', consider:

- narrow-complex tachycardia
    - sinus tachycardia
    - atrial tachycardia
    - atrial flutter
    - atrial fibrillation
    - AV re-entry tachycardia
    - AV nodal re-entry tachycardia
- broad-complex tachycardia
    - narrow-complex tachycardia with aberrant conduction
    - ventricular tachycardia
    - accelerated idioventricular rhythm
    - torsades de pointes.

## FURTHER READING

Details of Advanced Life Support guidelines, and training courses in resuscitation, can be obtained from the Resuscitation Council (UK) at: http://www.resus.org.uk/

Meek S, Morri F. ABC of clinical electrocardiography: Introduction. I – Leads, rate, rhythm, and cardiac axis. *Br Med J* 2002; **324**: 415–418.

In Chapters 7–9 we will be discussing the cardiac rhythms that you may encounter in everyday practice. To begin with, however, we will take an overview of how to approach the identification of a patient's cardiac rhythm. Following the step-by-step approach in this chapter will give you a firm foundation for tackling the problem of rhythm recognition.

To identify the cardiac rhythm with confidence you need to begin with a rhythm strip – a prolonged recording of the ECG from just one lead. Most ECG machines automatically include a rhythm strip at the bottom of a 12-lead ECG (Fig. 6.1). If your machine does not, make sure you have recorded one yourself. The machine may give you a choice about which of the 12 leads will appear as the rhythm strip – most commonly, lead II is selected as this tends to give the clearest view of P wave activity. However, sometimes it is necessary to select one of the other leads to gain a clearer picture of the rhythm.

The diagnosis of abnormal cardiac rhythms is not always easy, and some of the more complex arrhythmias can tax the skills of even the most experienced cardiologist. It is appropriate, therefore, to begin this chapter with the following warning:

**SEEK HELP**

If in doubt about a patient's cardiac rhythm, do not hesitate to seek the advice of a cardiologist.

This advice is particularly important if the patient is haemodynamically compromised by the arrhythmia, or if you are contemplating treatment of any kind.

There are many ways in which you can approach the identification of arrhythmias, and this is reflected in the numerous ways in which they can be categorized:

- regular versus irregular
- bradycardias versus tachycardias
- narrow complex versus broad complex
- supraventricular versus ventricular.

The common cardiac rhythms are listed in Table 6.1 and the following chapters contain a detailed description of each rhythm and its key characteristics, together with example ECGs. Let's begin, however, with a systematic strategy for working towards a rhythm diagnosis.

6 An approach to heart rhythms

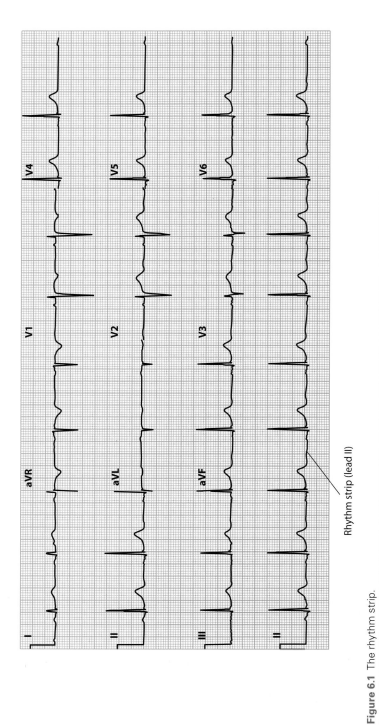

**Figure 6.1** The rhythm strip.

Key point:    • The standard lead used for the rhythm strip is lead II, but alternative leads can be selected if it helps to clarify the cardiac rhythm.

**Table 6.1** Cardiac rhythms

- SA nodal rhythms
  - sinus rhythm
  - sinus arrhythmia
  - sinus bradycardia
  - sinus tachycardia
  - sick sinus syndrome
- Atrial rhythms
  - atrial ectopic beats
  - atrial fibrillation
  - atrial flutter
  - atrial tachycardia
- Junctional rhythms
  - junctional ectopic beats
  - AV re-entry tachycardia (AVRT)
  - AV nodal re-entry tachycardia (AVNRT)
- Ventricular rhythms
  - ventricular ectopic beats
  - accelerated idioventricular rhythm
  - monomorphic ventricular tachycardia (VT)
  - polymorphic ventricular tachycardia ('torsades de pointes')
  - ventricular fibrillation (VF)
- Conduction problems
  - SA block
  - AV blocks
    - first-degree AV block
    - second-degree AV block
      - Mobitz type 1 AV block
      - Mobitz type 2 AV block
      - 2:1 AV block
    - third-degree AV block
  - Bundle branch and fascicular blocks
    - right bundle branch block
    - left bundle branch block
    - left anterior fascicular block
    - left posterior fascicular block
- Escape rhythms

## IDENTIFYING THE CARDIAC RHYTHM

When you analyse the cardiac rhythm, always keep in mind the two primary questions that you are trying to answer:

- Where does the impulse arise from?
  - sinoatrial (SA) node
  - atria
  - atrioventricular (AV) junction
  - ventricles

- How is the impulse conducted?
  - normal conduction
  - impaired conduction
  - accelerated conduction (e.g. WPW syndrome).

We will help you to narrow down the possible diagnoses with the following questions:

- How is the patient?
- Is ventricular activity present?
- What is the ventricular rate?
- Is the ventricular rhythm regular or irregular?
- Is the QRS complex width normal or broad?
- Is atrial activity present?
- How are atrial activity and ventricular activity related?

A similar approach to the ECG is used by the Resuscitation Council (UK) to train healthcare professionals in rhythm recognition. Attending an Advanced Life Support (ALS) course is an excellent way to improve your skills in cardiac rhythm recognition and, of course, in learning how to provide advanced life support. Contact details for the Resuscitation Council (UK) are provided at the end of this chapter (see *Further Reading*). If you live outside the UK, approach your local provider of ALS training for advice.

## HOW IS THE PATIENT?

Clinical context is all important in ECG interpretation, and so don't attempt to interpret an ECG rhythm without knowing the clinical context in which the ECG was recorded. Take the example of a rhythm strip that appears to show normal sinus rhythm. If it was recorded from a patient who is unconscious and pulseless, the diagnosis will be pulseless electrical activity (PEA), not sinus rhythm. Similarly, the presence of artefact on an ECG can be misread as an arrhythmia unless the clinical context is known. To avoid these problems:

- if you are interpreting an ECG that someone else has recorded, always insist on knowing the clinical details of the patient and the reason why it was recorded
- if you are recording an ECG that someone else will interpret later, always make a note of the clinical context at the top of the ECG to help with the interpretation (e.g. 'Patient experiencing chest pain at time of recording').

The clinical context will also help you decide how urgently to deal with an arrhythmia. When assessing a 'sick' patient, use the **ABCDE** approach:

- **Airway** – check for any evidence of airway obstruction
- **Breathing** – assess the patient's breathing, paying attention to respiratory rate, chest percussion and auscultation, and oxygenation
- **Circulation** – assess the patient's circulation, including pulse rate, blood pressure and capillary refill time
- **Disability** – assess level of consciousness and neurological status
- **Exposure** – ensure adequate exposure to permit a full examination.

As you assess a patient with an arrhythmia, be alert for so-called 'adverse features' which indicate haemodynamic instability:

- **shock** – as evidenced by hypotension (systolic blood pressure <90 mmHg), clamminess, sweating, pallor, confusion or reduced conscious level
- **syncope** – as a consequence of cerebral hypoperfusion
- **myocardial ischaemia** – indicated by ischaemic chest pain and/or ischaemic ECG changes (see Chapters 15 and 16)
- **heart failure** – pulmonary oedema, elevated jugular venous pressure, peripheral/ sacral oedema.

## IS VENTRICULAR ACTIVITY PRESENT?

Look at the ECG as a whole for the presence of electrical activity. If there is none, assess:

- the patient (do they have a pulse?)
- the electrodes (has something become disconnected?)
- the gain setting (is the gain setting on the monitor too low?).

If the patient is pulseless with no electrical activity evident on the ECG, they are in **asystole** and appropriate emergency action must be taken – see page 85 for more details. Beware of diagnosing asystole in the presence of a *completely* flat ECG trace – there should usually be some baseline drift present. A completely flat line usually means an electrode has become disconnected – check the electrodes (and, of course, the patient) carefully when making your diagnosis.

P waves may appear on their own (for a short time) after the onset of ventricular asystole. The presence of 'P waves only' on the ECG is important to recognize, as the patient may respond to emergency pacing manoeuvres such as percussion pacing, transcutaneous pacing or temporary transvenous pacing.

If QRS complexes are present, move on to the next question.

## WHAT IS THE VENTRICULAR RATE?

Ventricular activity is represented on the ECG by QRS complexes. The methods for determining the ventricular rate are discussed in Chapter 5. Once you have calculated the ventricular rate, you will be able to classify the rhythm as:

- bradycardia (<60 beats/min)
- normal (60–100 beats/min)
- tachycardia (>100 beats/min).

## IS THE VENTRICULAR RHYTHM REGULAR OR IRREGULAR?

Having determined the ventricular rate, go on to assess regularity. Look at the spacing between QRS complexes – is it the same throughout the rhythm strip? Irregularity can be subtle, so it is useful to measure out the distance between each QRS complex. One way to do this is to place a piece of paper alongside the rhythm strip and make a mark on it next to every QRS complex. By moving the marked paper up and down along the rhythm strip, you can soon see if the gaps between the QRS complexes are the same or vary. Once you have assessed the regularity, you will be able to classify the ventricular rhythm as:

- regular (equal spacing between QRS complexes)
- irregular (variable spacing between QRS complexes).

Table 6.2 lists the causes of regular and irregular cardiac rhythms.

If the rhythm is irregular, it is helpful to try to characterize the degree of irregularity. **Atrial fibrillation**, for example, is a totally chaotic rhythm with no discernible pattern to the QRS complexes (page 59). **Sinus arrhythmia**, by comparison, shows a cyclical variation in ventricular rate that is not chaotic but has a clear periodicity to it, coinciding with the patient's breathing movements (page 54).

In **intermittent AV block**, if an impulse is blocked *en route* to the ventricles as a result of a conduction problem, the corresponding QRS complex will fail to appear where expected and the beat will be 'missed' (see Fig. 9.4). The degree of irregularity will depend upon the nature of the conduction problem – the block of impulses may be predictable, in which case there will be a 'regular irregularity', or unpredictable.

Similarly, **ectopic beats** may occur in a predictable manner or unpredictably, giving rise to regular or irregular irregularities accordingly. In ventricular bigeminy, for example, a ventricular ectopic beat arises after each normal QRS complex, leading to a 'regular irregularity' of the ventricular rhythm (Fig. 8.2).

**Table 6.2** Regular and irregular cardiac rhythms

- Regular rhythms
  - sinus rhythm
  - sinus bradycardia
  - sinus tachycardia
  - atrial flutter (if constant AV block, e.g. 2:1)
  - atrial tachycardia
  - AV re-entry tachycardia (AVRT)
  - AV nodal re-entry tachycardia (AVNRT)
  - accelerated idioventricular rhythm
  - monomorphic ventricular tachycardia (VT)
  - polymorphic ventricular tachycardia ('torsades de pointes')
  - second-degree AV block
    - 2:1 AV block
  - third-degree AV block (if regular escape rhythm)
- Irregular rhythms
  - sinus arrhythmia (rate varies with respiration)
  - ectopic beats (atrial, junctional, ventricular)
  - atrial fibrillation
  - atrial flutter (if variable AV block)
  - sinus arrest and SA block
  - second-degree AV block
    - Mobitz type 1 AV block
    - Mobitz type 2 AV block

# IS THE QRS COMPLEX WIDTH NORMAL OR BROAD?

The width of the QRS complex can provide valuable clues about the origin of the cardiac rhythm. By answering this question, you will have narrowed down the origin of the impulse to one half of the heart. Ventricular rhythms are generated within the ventricular myocardium; supraventricular rhythms are generated anywhere up to (and including) the AV junction (Fig. 6.2).

Normally, the ventricles are depolarized via the His–Purkinje system, a network of rapidly conducting fibres that run throughout the ventricular myocardium. As a result, the ventricles are normally completely depolarized within 0.12 s, and the corresponding QRS complex on the ECG is less than 3 small squares wide.

However, if there is a problem with conduction within the ventricles, such as a block of part of the His–Purkinje system (as seen in left or right bundle branch block), depolarization has to spread directly from myocyte to myocyte instead. This takes longer, and so the QRS complex becomes wider than 3 small squares. This is also the case if the impulse has arisen within the ventricles (instead of coming via the AV node), as in the case of a ventricular ectopic beat or in VT. If an impulse does not pass through the AV node, it cannot use the His–Purkinje conduction system. Once again, it must travel from myocyte to myocyte, prolonging the process of depolarization.

This allows us to use the width of the QRS complex to try to determine how the ventricles were depolarized. If the QRS complex is narrow (<3 small squares), the ventricles must have been rapidly depolarized by an impulse that came through the AV node – the only way into the His–Purkinje system. The patient is then said to have a **supraventricular rhythm** (arising from above the ventricles).

If the QRS complex is broad (>3 small squares), there are two possible explanations:

1. The impulse may have arisen from within the ventricles and thus been unable to travel via the His–Purkinje system (**ventricular rhythm**).

2. The impulse may have arisen from above the ventricles but not been able to use all the His–Purkinje system because of a conduction problem (**supraventricular rhythm with aberrant conduction**).

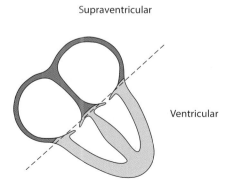

Supraventricular

Ventricular

**Figure 6.2** Supraventricular versus ventricular rhythms.

Key point:  • Supraventricular applies to any structure above the ventricles (and electrically distinct from them).

**Table 6.3** Broad-complex versus narrow-complex rhythms. Only supraventricular rhythms with normal conduction can gain access to the His–Purkinje system to depolarize the ventricles rapidly.

| Rhythm origin | Rhythm conduction | QRS complex |
|---|---|---|
| Supraventricular | Normal | Narrow |
| Supraventricular | Aberrant (e.g. bundle branch block) | Broad |
| Ventricular | Myocyte-to-myocyte | Broad |

This is summarized in Table 6.3.

Trying to distinguish between ventricular rhythms and supraventricular rhythms with aberrant conduction can be difficult, particularly if the patient is tachycardic and there is concern that the rhythm is VT. The distinction between VT and SVT is discussed specifically on page 86.

## IS ATRIAL ACTIVITY PRESENT?

Atrial electrical activity can take several forms, which can be grouped into four categories:

- P waves (atrial depolarization)
- flutter waves (atrial flutter)
- fibrillation waves (atrial fibrillation)
- unclear activity.

The presence of **P waves** indicates atrial depolarization. This does not mean that the depolarization necessarily started at the SA node, however. P waves will appear during atrial depolarization regardless of where it originated – it is the *orientation* of the P waves that tells you where the depolarization originated (Chapter 7). Upright P waves in lead II suggest that atrial depolarization originated in or near the SA node. Inverted P waves suggest an origin closer to, or within, the AV node (Fig. 11.4).

**Flutter waves** are seen in atrial flutter at a rate of 300/min, creating a sawtooth base-line of atrial activity (Fig. 7.8). This can be made more readily apparent by manoeu-vres that transiently block the AV node (page 66).

**Fibrillation waves** are seen in AF and correspond to random, chaotic atrial impulses occurring at a rate of around 400–600/min (Fig. 7.7). This leads to a chaotic, low-amplitude baseline of atrial activity.

The nature of the atrial activity may be **unclear**. This may be because P waves are 'hidden' within the QRS complexes, as is often the case during AV nodal re-entry tachycardia. In such cases atrial depolarization *is* taking place, but its electri-cal 'signature' on the ECG cannot easily be seen because the simultaneous, larger amplitude, QRS complex hides it. Atrial activity may also be absent in, for example, sinus arrest or SA block, in which case the atria may be electrically silent.

## HOW ARE ATRIAL ACTIVITY AND VENTRICULAR ACTIVITY RELATED?

Having examined the activity of the atria and of the ventricles, the final task is to determine how the two are related. Normally an impulse from the atria goes on to depolarize the ventricles, leading to a 1:1 relationship between P waves and QRS complexes. However, impulses from the atria may sometimes fail to reach the ventricles, or the ventricles may generate their own impulses independent of the atria.

If every QRS complex is associated with a P wave, this indicates that the atria and ventricles are being activated by a common source. This is usually, but not necessarily, the SA node (e.g. AV junctional rhythms will also depolarize both atria and ventricles).

If there are more P waves than QRS complexes, conduction between atria and ventricles is being either partly blocked (with only some impulses getting through) or completely blocked (with the ventricles having developed their own escape rhythm). Conduction problems are discussed further in Chapter 9.

More QRS complexes than P waves indicates AV dissociation (p. 135), with the ventricles operating independently of the atria and at a higher rate (Fig. 12.10).

Always bear in mind that the P wave may be difficult or even impossible to discern clearly. Therefore, it can sometimes be difficult to say conclusively that atrial activity is absent.

## DETERMINING THE CARDIAC RHYTHM

Using the seven questions above, you now have a 'toolkit' with which to tackle the diagnosis of cardiac rhythms. As you read about supraventricular rhythms, ventricular rhythms and conduction problems in the next three chapters, think about these seven questions and how they relate to each of the rhythms described. Each rhythm has its own set of ECG characteristics, and by assessing the ECG in a methodical manner you will quickly learn how to distinguish between them.

There are a handful of rhythms that you should learn by rote so that you can recognize them without hesitation in an emergency – these are the **cardiac arrest rhythms** (ventricular fibrillation, ventricular tachycardia, asystole and pulseless electrical activity), which are also discussed further in the following chapters.

## SUMMARY

When assessing the cardiac rhythm, consider the following:

- SA nodal rhythms
  - sinus rhythm
  - sinus arrhythmia
  - sinus bradycardia
  - sinus tachycardia
  - sick sinus syndrome
- atrial rhythms
  - atrial ectopic beats
  - atrial fibrillation
  - atrial flutter
  - atrial tachycardia

*(Continued)*

(*Continued*)
- junctional rhythms
  - junctional ectopic beats
  - AV re-entry tachycardia (AVRT)
  - AV nodal re-entry tachycardia (AVNRT)
- ventricular rhythms
  - ventricular ectopic beats
  - accelerated idioventricular rhythm
  - monomorphic ventricular tachycardia (VT)
  - polymorphic ventricular tachycardia ('torsades de pointes')
  - ventricular fibrillation (VF)
- conduction problems
  - SA block
  - AV blocks
    - first-degree AV block
    - second-degree AV block
      - Mobitz type 1 AV block
      - Mobitz type 2 AV block
      - 2:1 AV block
    - third-degree AV block
  - bundle branch and fascicular blocks
    - right bundle branch block
    - left bundle branch block
    - left anterior fascicular block
    - left posterior fascicular block
- escape rhythms.

To identify the rhythm, ask yourself the following questions:

*1. Where does the impulse arise from?*
- SA node
- atria
- AV junction
- ventricles.

*2. How is the impulse conducted?*
- normal conduction
- impaired conduction
- accelerated conduction (e.g. WPW syndrome).

## FURTHER READING

Details of Advanced Life Support guidelines, and training courses in resuscitation, can be obtained from the Resuscitation Council (UK) at: http://www.resus.org.uk/

Wellens HJJ. Ventricular tachycardia: diagnosis of broad QRS complex tachycardia. *Heart* 2001; **86**: 579–585.

Whinnett ZI, Sohaib SMA, Davies DW. Diagnosis and management of supraventricular tachycardia. *BMJ* 2012; **345**: e7769.

# CHAPTER 7

# Supraventricular rhythms

Supraventricular rhythms are those which arise above the level of the ventricles, i.e. from the sinoatrial (SA) node, the atria or the atrioventricular (AV) node. This includes normal rhythms (sinus rhythm, sinus arrhythmia), abnormal rhythms (e.g. atrial fibrillation, atrial flutter, etc.), and rhythms which may or may not be 'normal' depending upon the clinical context (e.g. sinus tachycardia). All of these are discussed in this chapter.

The supraventricular rhythms we will consider are:

- sinus rhythm
- sinus arrhythmia
- sinus bradycardia
- sinus tachycardia
- sick sinus syndrome
- atrial ectopic beats
- atrial fibrillation
- atrial flutter
- atrial tachycardia
  - focal atrial tachycardia
  - multifocal atrial tachycardia
- atrioventricular re-entry tachycardia (AVRT)
- atrioventricular nodal re-entry tachycardia (AVNRT).

## SINUS RHYTHM

Sinus rhythm is the normal cardiac rhythm, in which the SA node acts as the natural pacemaker, discharging at a rate of 60–100/min (Fig. 7.1). The characteristic features of sinus rhythm are:

- heart rate is 60–100/min
- P wave morphology is normal (e.g. upright in lead II and inverted in lead aVR)
- every P wave is followed by a QRS complex.

If the patient is in sinus rhythm, move on to check whether there might be any conduction problems (Chapter 9) and then determine the cardiac axis (Chapter 10) before assessing the rest of the ECG step-by-step (Chapters 11–18). If not, continue reading this chapter to diagnose the rhythm.

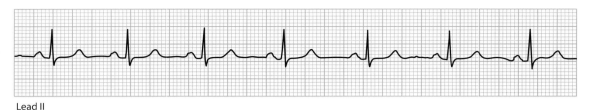

Lead II

**Figure 7.1** Normal sinus rhythm.

Key point: • The heart rate is 75/min, the P waves are upright (lead II) and every P wave is followed by a QRS complex.

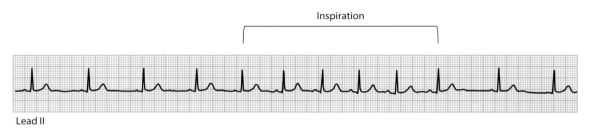

Lead II

**Figure 7.2** Physiological sinus arrhythmia.

Key point: • The heart rate increases during inspiration, the P waves are upright (lead II) and every P wave is followed by a QRS complex.

## SINUS ARRHYTHMIA

Sinus arrhythmia is the variation in heart rate that is seen during inspiration and expiration (Fig. 7.2). The characteristic features of sinus arrhythmia are:

- the heart rate varies with respiration
- during *inspiration*, the heart rate *increases* as a reflex response to the increased volume of blood returning to the heart
- during *expiration*, the heart rate *decreases* as a reflex response to the decreased volume of blood returning to the heart
- P wave morphology is normal (e.g. upright in lead II and inverted in lead aVR)
- every P wave is followed by a QRS complex.

Sinus arrhythmia is uncommon after the age of 40 years. Sinus arrhythmia is harmless and no investigations or treatment are necessary.

## SINUS BRADYCARDIA

Sinus bradycardia is sinus rhythm with a heart rate of less than 60/min (Fig. 7.3). The characteristic features of sinus bradycardia are:

- the heart rate is *less than* 60/min
- P wave morphology is normal (e.g. upright in lead II and inverted in lead aVR)
- every P wave is followed by a QRS complex.

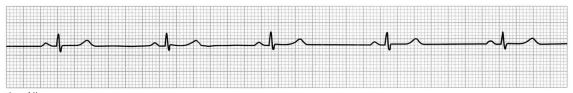

Lead II

**Figure 7.3** Sinus bradycardia.

Key point:  • The heart rate is 46/min, the P waves are upright (lead II) and every P wave is followed by a QRS complex.

It is unusual for sinus bradycardia to be slower than 40/min. Sinus bradycardia can be a normal finding, e.g. in athletes during sleep. However, always consider the following possible causes:

- drugs (e.g. digoxin, beta blockers – including beta blocker eye drops)
- ischaemic heart disease and myocardial infarction
- hypothyroidism
- hypothermia
- electrolyte abnormalities
- obstructive jaundice
- uraemia
- raised intracranial pressure
- sick sinus syndrome.

If the sinus bradycardia is severe, escape beats and escape rhythms may occur (Chapter 9). The management of bradycardia (of any cause) is discussed in Chapter 5.

## SINUS TACHYCARDIA

Sinus tachycardia is sinus rhythm with a heart rate of greater than 100/min (Fig. 7.4). The characteristic features of sinus tachycardia are:

- the heart rate is *greater than* 100/min
- P wave morphology is normal (e.g. upright in lead II and inverted in lead aVR)
- every P wave is followed by a QRS complex.

It is unusual for sinus tachycardia to exceed 180/min, except in fit athletes. At this heart rate, it may be difficult to differentiate the P waves from the T waves, so the rhythm can be mistaken for an AV nodal re-entry tachycardia (p. 73).

Physiological causes of sinus tachycardia include anything that stimulates the sympathetic nervous system – anxiety, pain, fear, fever or exercise. Always consider the following causes as well:

- drugs, e.g. adrenaline, atropine, salbutamol (do not forget inhalers and nebulizers), caffeine and alcohol
- ischaemic heart disease and acute myocardial infarction
- heart failure
- pulmonary embolism

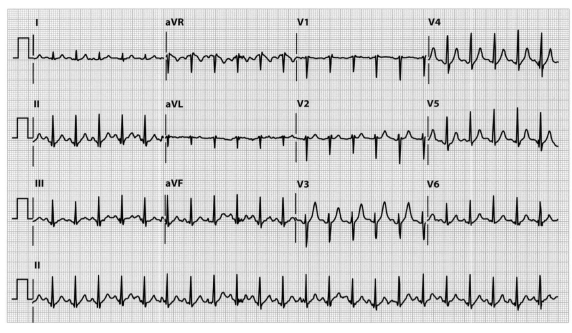

**Figure 7.4** Sinus tachycardia.

Key point:    • The heart rate is 136/min, the P waves have a normal orientation in each lead, and every P wave is followed by a QRS complex.

- fluid loss
- anaemia
- hyperthyroidism.

The management of sinus tachycardia is that of the cause. When a patient has an **appropriate** tachycardia (e.g. compensating for low blood pressure, such as in fluid loss), the tachycardia is helping to maintain the patient's blood pressure and so slowing it with beta blockers can lead to disastrous decompensation. It is the underlying problem that needs addressing. However, if the sinus tachycardia is **inappropriate**, as in anxiety or hyperthyroidism, then the tachycardia is counterproductive and using drug treatment (e.g. beta blockers) to slow the tachycardia may be helpful.

  **WARNING**

In sinus tachycardia, never attempt to slow the heart rate until you have established the cause.

*Persistent* 'sinus tachycardia' should lead to suspicion that the diagnosis may be incorrect – both atrial flutter and atrial tachycardia can, on casual inspection, be mistaken for sinus tachycardia. However, persistent 'inappropriate' sinus tachycardia is recognized as a clinical entity, referring to a persistent increase in daytime resting heart rate (>100/min) which is out of proportion to any clinical factors, and with an excessive increase in heart rate on physical activity. P wave morphology is normal. The condition is poorly understood, but it may result

7 Supraventricular rhythms

from enhanced automaticity within the SA node or from autonomic dysfunction. Inappropriate sinus tachycardia can be treated with rate-controlling drugs (such as beta blockers) or, in severe symptomatic cases, electrophysiological modification/ablation of the SA node. Careful exclusion of any underlying physiological factors (e.g. hyperthyroidism) is essential.

## SICK SINUS SYNDROME

As the name suggests, sick sinus syndrome is a collection of impulse generation and conduction problems related to dysfunction of the sinus node. Any, or all, of the following problems may be seen in a patient with the syndrome:

- sinus bradycardia
- sinus tachycardia
- sinus arrest
- SA block.

**Sinus bradycardia** and **sinus tachycardia** have already been described. The sinus node is normally a very reliable pacemaker. However, in **sinus arrest**, it sometimes fails to discharge on time – looking at a rhythm strip, a P wave will suddenly fail to appear in the expected place, and there is a gap, of variable length, until the sinus node fires and a P wave appears, or a junctional escape beat is generated by a 'safety net' subsidiary pacemaker in the AV junction (Fig. 11.3). In sick sinus syndrome, it's not unusual to observe a prolonged pause after an episode of atrial tachyarrhythmia.

In an **SA block**, the sinus node depolarizes as normal, but the impulse fails to reach the atria. A P wave fails to appear in the expected place, but the next one usually appears exactly where it is expected (Fig. 9.2).

If the sinus bradycardia is severe, or if sinus arrest or SA block is prolonged, escape rhythms (p. 102) may occur. Sick sinus syndrome may also coexist with:

- atrial fibrillation (p. 59)
- atrial flutter (p. 64)
- atrial tachycardia (p. 66).

The association of sick sinus syndrome with paroxysmal tachycardias is called **tachycardia–bradycardia (or 'tachy-brady') syndrome**.

Sick sinus syndrome, and the associated tachy-brady syndrome, may cause symptoms of dizziness, fainting and palpitation. The commonest cause of sick sinus syndrome is degeneration and fibrosis of the sinoatrial node. Other causes to consider are:

- ischaemic heart disease
- drugs (e.g. beta blockers, digoxin, quinidine)
- cardiomyopathy
- amyloidosis
- myocarditis.

The diagnosis usually requires ambulatory ECG monitoring (Chapter 21).

Asymptomatic patients do not require treatment. Patients with symptoms need consideration for a permanent pacemaker (Chapter 20). This is particularly important if they also have paroxysmal tachycardias that require anti-arrhythmic drugs (which can worsen the episodes of bradycardia). Paroxysmal tachycardias that arise as escape rhythms in response to episodes of bradycardia may also improve as a consequence of pacing. Referral to a cardiologist is therefore recommended.

## ATRIAL ECTOPIC BEATS

Ectopic beats appear *earlier* than expected and can arise from any region of the heart (usually being classified into atrial, AV junctional and ventricular ectopics). Atrial ectopic beats are also called atrial extrasystoles, atrial premature complexes (APCs), atrial premature beats (APBs) or premature atrial contractions (PACs).

Atrial ectopic beats are identified by a P wave that appears earlier than expected and has a different shape to the normal P waves (Fig. 7.5). Although atrial ectopic beats will usually be conducted to the ventricles and give rise to a QRS complex, occasionally they may encounter a refractory AV node and fail to be conducted.

AV junctional ectopic beats will activate the ventricles, giving rise to a QRS complex earlier than expected (Fig. 7.6). They may also retrogradely activate the atria

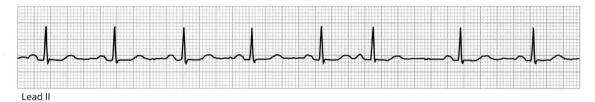

Lead II

**Figure 7.5**  Atrial ectopic beat.

Key points:  • After five normal sinus beats, the sixth beat is an atrial ectopic.
  • It occurs earlier than expected, and the shape of the P wave is different to that of the normal P waves in sinus rhythm, indicating an origin in a different part of the atria.

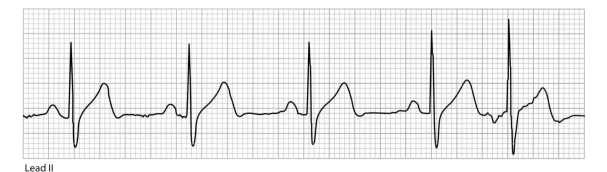

Lead II

**Figure 7.6**  AV junctional ectopic beat.

Key points:  • After four normal sinus beats, the fifth beat is an AV junctional ectopic.
  • It occurs earlier than expected, and the P wave is inverted, indicating an origin low down in the atria, at the AV junction.

to cause an inverted P wave. Whether the P wave occurs before, during or after the QRS complex simply depends on whether the electrical impulse reaches the atria or ventricles first.

Atrial and AV junctional ectopic beats are a common finding in normal individuals and do not usually require specific treatment unless they cause troublesome symptoms, in which case beta blockers can reduce their frequency.

## ATRIAL FIBRILLATION

Atrial fibrillation (AF) is a common and important arrhythmia, affecting 1.5–2% of people in the developed world, and is associated with an increased risk of stroke and heart failure. Owing to the aging population, the prevalence of AF is predicted to at least double over the next 50 years.

The basis of AF is rapid, chaotic depolarization occurring throughout the atria as a consequence of multiple 'wavelets' of activation. No P waves are seen and the ECG baseline consists of low-amplitude oscillations (fibrillation or 'f' waves). Although around 400–600 impulses reach the AV node every minute, only some will be transmitted to the ventricles. The ventricular rate is typically fast (100–180/min), although the rate can be normal or even slow. Transmission of the atrial impulses through the AV node is erratic, making the ventricular (QRS complex) rhythm 'irregularly irregular'.

Thus, the characteristic ECG features of AF are:

- absence of distinct P waves
- irregularly irregular ventricular rhythm (Fig. 7.7).

Five categories of AF are recognized:

- **first-diagnosed AF** – namely, patients presenting in AF for the first time
- **paroxysmal AF** – self-terminating episodes of AF, typically lasting <48 h although they can last up to 7 days
- **persistent AF** – an episode of continuous AF lasting >7 days or requiring cardioversion
- **long-standing persistent AF** – where AF has been present for at least one year, but there is still an aim to restore sinus rhythm
- **permanent AF** – continuous AF where the arrhythmia is 'accepted' and there is no plan to restore sinus rhythm.

Patients can progress between categories – for instance, a patient whose AF is initially paroxysmal may eventually develop persistent AF which, if sinus rhythm

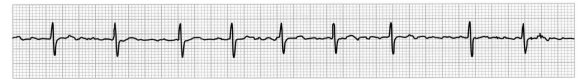

Lead II

**Figure 7.7** Atrial fibrillation.

Key point:    • The ventricular rhythm is irregularly irregular, with an absence of distinct P waves.

is not restored, will later become long-standing persistent AF, and if the AF is ultimately 'accepted' then it is said to be permanent.

## Clinical assessment

AF can be asymptomatic, but many patients will experience one or more of the following symptoms:

- fast, irregular palpitation
- breathlessness
- fatigue.

The loss of co-ordinated atrial contraction (atrial 'kick') as a result of AF can be particularly troublesome, leading to a drop in cardiac output of 5–15%. The severity of AF symptoms can be expressed in terms of an EHRA (European Heart Rhythm Association) score (Table 7.1). Thromboembolism is an important risk in AF and may also be a presenting feature, such as transient ischaemic attack, stroke or peripheral embolism. There may also be symptoms related to an underlying cause for the AF, such as angina or thyrotoxicosis.

Examination of the patient will reveal an irregularly irregular pulse, often with a rapid ventricular rate. The examination should identify any consequence of the AF (such as heart failure) and any causative or contributing factors (e.g. hypertension, valvular heart disease). The causes of AF are listed in Table 7.2. Where a cause cannot be identified, the AF is described as idiopathic or 'lone' AF.

Investigations should include a 12-lead ECG and blood tests to check electrolytes and renal function, thyroid function tests and a full blood count. Patients should be screened for diabetes. Echocardiography is used to screen for structural heart disease. Where appropriate, investigations for coronary artery disease may also be required.

**Table 7.1** EHRA classification of AF symptoms

| EHRA class | Severity of AF symptoms |
|---|---|
| I | Asymptomatic |
| II | Mild symptoms (not affecting daily activities) |
| III | Severe symptoms (affecting daily activities) |
| IV | Disabling symptoms (unable to undertake daily activities) |

**Table 7.2** Causes of atrial fibrillation

- Hypertension
- Ischaemic heart disease
- Valvular heart disease
- Cardiomyopathies
- Myocarditis
- Atrial septal defect and other congenital heart disease
- Hyperthyroidism
- Alcohol
- Pulmonary embolism
- Pneumonia
- Cardiac surgery

Key issues to consider in managing patients with AF are:

- reducing stroke risk
- ventricular rate control
- rhythm control.

## Reducing stroke risk

The presence of AF increases a patient's stroke risk five-fold, and one in five strokes occurs as a result of AF. Strokes that occur in AF are more likely to be disabling or fatal. Reducing stroke risk in AF is therefore important, and the approach can be summarized as follows:

- for patients with valvular AF (including rheumatic valve disease and prosthetic valves), anticoagulation with warfarin is recommended for all, unless there are contraindications
- for those with non-valvular AF, antithrombotic therapy is recommended for all, except in those patients who are at low risk (aged <65 years and lone AF), or with contraindications.

The risk of thromboembolism in non-valvular AF can be assessed using the $CHA_2DS_2$-VASc scoring system, where the risk factors for thromboembolic events are scored as follows:

- **C** – congestive heart failure (1 point)
- **H** – hypertension (1 point)
- **A** – age ≥75 years (2 points)
- **D** – diabetes mellitus (1 point)
- **S** – previous stroke or TIA (2 points)
- **V** – vascular disease (1 point)
- **A** – age 65–74 years (1 point)
- **Sc** – sex category (1 point if female)

Patients can score between 0 and 9 points. For those with a score of 0, no antithrombotic therapy is recommended. With a score of 1 or more, oral anticoagulant therapy (using warfarin or one of the novel oral anticoagulants, such as dabigatran) is recommended. However female patients who are aged <65 years and have lone AF (i.e. those who have a $CHA_2DS_2$-VASc score of 1 only as a result of female gender) are low-risk and do not require an oral anticoagulant.

Before recommending oral anticoagulants, patients should also be assessed for potential bleeding risk using the HAS-BLED score:

- **H** – hypertension
- **A** – abnormal renal/liver function (1 point each)
- **S** – stroke
- **B** – bleeding tendency or predisposition
- **L** – labile INR if on warfarin
- **E** – elderly
- **D** – drugs (e.g. aspirin, NSAIDs)/alcohol concomitantly (1 point each)

A HAS-BLED score ≥3 indicates a 'high risk' for bleeding, and antithrombotic therapy should be used with caution and with regular review. The HAS-BLED score is particularly helpful in identifying modifiable risk factors for bleeding, which might then be managed to reduce the risk.

If patients refuse oral anticoagulants, antiplatelet therapy (using aspirin 75–100 mg plus clopidogrel 75 mg daily or, less effectively, aspirin 75–325 mg daily) may be considered as an alternative. However, antiplatelet therapy is not as effective as anticoagulant therapy, and the risk of major bleeding is broadly similar to that with oral anticoagulant therapy.

> **THE LEFT ATRIAL APPENDAGE AND STROKE RISK**
>
> The principal (but not only) site of thrombus formation in AF is the left atrial appendage, a small pouch or 'pocket' that is part of the left atrium and in which blood can 'stagnate' and clot. For patients with a high stroke risk but contraindications to long-term anticoagulation, one option is percutaneous occlusion/closure of the left atrial appendage, which is performed as an interventional procedure using a specialized closure device. For patients who are undergoing heart surgery, a further option is surgical excision of the left atrial appendage.

## Ventricular rate control

Commonly used drugs for ventricular rate control include beta blockers and non-dihydropyridine calcium channel blockers (verapamil or diltiazem). Digoxin is good for rate control at rest but is poor at rate control during exercise. Although amiodarone is effective for rate control, it does carry a risk of significant adverse effects and should generally be avoided for long-term rate control unless safer alternatives cannot be used.

Rate control is the preferred strategy (instead of rhythm control) in elderly patients and those with minimal symptoms (EHRA class I). Initially, a lenient rate control strategy can be adopted, aiming for a resting ventricular rate <110/min. If patients remain symptomatic, a stricter rate control strategy can be used, aiming for a resting heart rate <80/min (with a heart rate <110/min during moderate exercise).

If drug therapy cannot attain satisfactory rate control in AF, and restoration of sinus rhythm cannot be achieved, an alternative strategy is to undertake ablation of the AV node plus permanent pacing. This places the patient in complete heart block, and they are then pacemaker-dependent. While this is an effective means of achieving control over their ventricular rate, the patient's atria nonetheless continue to fibrillate which means they will still suffer from the haemodynamic consequences of a loss of atrial 'kick' (p. 60) and will still require antithrombotic therapy (where appropriate).

## Rhythm control

Patients with symptomatic AF (EHRA class II–IV) despite adequate ventricular rate control should be considered for a rhythm control strategy, where the aim is to restore and maintain sinus rhythm.

### Cardioverting to sinus rhythm

For those with recent onset AF and who are haemodynamically unstable, urgent electrical cardioversion is advised. Similarly, patients who are stable and who present within 48 h of the onset of AF can have urgent electrical cardioversion. In both cases, anticoagulant cover using intravenous unfractionated heparin is advised initially, followed by a minimum of four weeks' oral anticoagulation (unless the patient is aged <65 years and has had 'lone' AF).

If a patient presents within 48 h of the onset of AF but would prefer not to undergo electrical cardioversion, an alternative is pharmacological ('chemical') cardioversion:

- if there is no structural heart disease – intravenous flecainide, ibutilide, propafenone or vernakalant are first-line options, and intravenous amiodarone is a second-line option

- if there is moderate structural heart disease – intravenous ibutilide (unless there is left ventricular hypertrophy ≥1.4 cm) or vernakalant (unless there is moderate or severe heart failure, aortic stenosis, acute coronary syndrome or hypotension; caution is required in mild heart failure) are first-line options, and intravenous amiodarone is a second-line option

- if there is severe structural heart disease – intravenous amiodarone is the first-line option.

The need for appropriate anticoagulation is the same whether cardioversion is undertaken electrically or pharmacologically.

For patients who have been in AF for >48 h, a transoesophageal echocardiogram can be performed to rule out intracardiac thrombus before undertaking electrical cardioversion. If a transoesophageal echocardiogram is not possible, the patient should be therapeutically anticoagulated for a minimum of three weeks before any attempt is made at electrical cardioversion.

---

### ELECTRICAL CARDIOVERSION FOR AF

Although electrical cardioversion for AF is often initially successful in restoring sinus rhythm, the arrhythmia frequently recurs. Long-term success is more likely if patients have been in AF for only a short time and if there is no structural heart disease.

Patients must be 'nil by mouth' on the day of the procedure as they will require general anaesthesia. Check their electrolyte levels and, where appropriate, their international normalized ratio (INR). The plasma potassium level should be ≥4 mmol/L. If the patient is taking digoxin and there is a possibility of digoxin toxicity (suggested by symptoms, ECG findings, high dosage or renal impairment), check the patient's digoxin level.

Set the defibrillator to synchronized mode and start at an energy level of 100–120 J (biphasic), increasing to 200 J as appropriate. In atrial flutter, lower energy levels may be successful. Monophasic defibrillators will require higher energy levels.

If cardioversion is successful, continue anticoagulation and review the patient after four weeks. Anticoagulation may be discontinued at that point, although it should be continued if there are risk factors for stroke or AF recurrence, or thrombus is present.

---

## Maintaining sinus rhythm

Once a patient is back in sinus rhythm, and you wish to reduce the risk of future paroxysms of AF, the following longer-term oral treatment options can be considered:

- if there is minimal or no structural heart disease, first-line options include sotalol, flecainide, dronedarone, and propafenone; the second-line option is amiodarone

- if there is significant structural heart disease, ensure the underlying condition is effectively treated, and consider the following:
  - if there is heart failure, amiodarone is the preferred option
  - if there is coronary heart disease, sotalol is the preferred option, with dronedarone second-line and amiodarone third-line
  - if there is hypertensive heart disease with left ventricular hypertrophy, dronedarone is the preferred option, with amiodarone second-line.

## Catheter ablation of AF

Catheter ablation for AF usually involves electrical isolation of some or all of the pulmonary veins and is more effective than drug therapy in maintaining sinus rhythm, but does involve an invasive electrophysiological procedure with its attendant risks.

Catheter ablation is indicated for patients with paroxysmal AF who have symptomatic recurrences on drug therapy, and is also a reasonable first-line option for patients with paroxysmal AF who prefer to avoid long-term anti-arrhythmic drug treatment.

## ATRIAL FLUTTER

Atrial flutter is often considered to be a subtype of atrial tachycardia (p. 66) and is characterized by a macro re-entry circuit, typically within the right atrium and involving the cavotricuspid isthmus (CTI-dependent or Type I flutter). Less commonly, other forms of flutter are seen that do not involve the CTI (non-CTI-dependent or Type II flutter). These usually occur in relation to an area of scar tissue in the atria, often in the context of prior cardiac surgery.

In the commonest form of atrial flutter, it takes about 0.2 s for the impulse to complete a circuit in the right atrium (in most cases moving in a counterclockwise direction), each time giving rise to a wave of depolarization and a flutter wave on the ECG. There are thus about five flutter waves every second, and so around 300 every minute (Fig. 7.8).

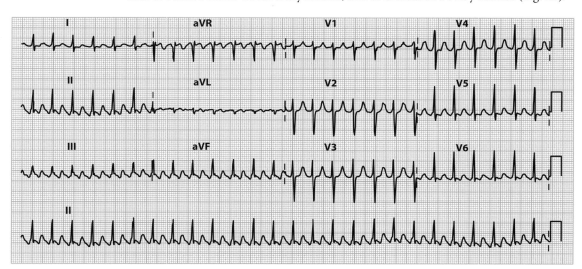

**Figure 7.8** Atrial flutter.

Key point:
- There is a 'sawtooth' pattern of atrial activity, with an atrial rate of 300/min and a ventricular rate of 150/min (indicating 2:1 AV block).

In atrial flutter the atrial rate is usually 250–350/min and often almost exactly 300/min. The AV node cannot normally keep up with such a high atrial rate and AV block occurs. This is most commonly 2:1 block, where only alternate atrial impulses get through the AV node to initiate a QRS complex, although 3:1, 4:1 (Fig. 7.9) or variable degrees of block (Fig. 7.10) are also seen.

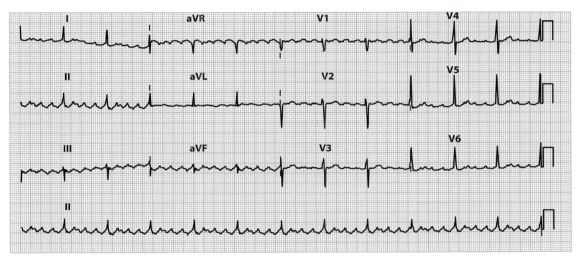

**Figure 7.9** Atrial flutter.

Key point:    • There is a 'sawtooth' pattern of atrial activity, with an atrial rate of 288/min and a ventricular rate of 72/min (indicating 4:1 AV block).

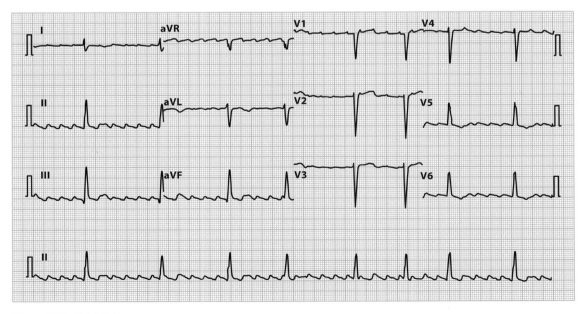

**Figure 7.10** Atrial flutter.

Key points:    • There is a 'sawtooth' pattern of atrial activity, with an atrial rate of 250/min and a ventricular rate of 48/min.
• The ventricular rhythm is irregular, indicating variable AV block.

7 Supraventricular rhythms

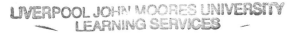

Thus, the ventricular rate is less than the atrial rate, and is often 150, 100 or 75/min. You should always suspect atrial flutter with 2:1 block when a patient has a regular tachycardia with a ventricular rate of about 150/min.

The rapid atrial rate gives a characteristic 'sawtooth' appearance to the baseline of the ECG, made up of flutter or 'F' waves. This can be made more apparent by carotid sinus massage or by giving adenosine. This will not terminate the atrial flutter, but will increase the degree of AV block, making the baseline easier to see by reducing the number of QRS complexes. Carotid sinus massage should be performed with the patient supine and with the neck slightly extended. Do not perform carotid sinus massage if carotid bruits are present, or if there is a history of cerebral thromboembolism. Massage the carotid artery on one side of the neck, medial to the sternomastoid muscle, for 5 s. The technique can be repeated, if necessary, on the opposite side after waiting for 1 min. The ECG must be monitored continuously throughout the procedure.

Thus, the characteristic features of atrial flutter are:

- atrial rate around 300/min
- 'sawtooth' baseline
- AV block (commonly 2:1, but can be 3:1, 4:1 or variable).

The predisposing factors for atrial flutter are similar to those for AF (see Table 7.2). Although beta blockers, verapamil or digoxin can be used simply to control the ventricular response, it is preferable to aim to restore sinus rhythm. Atrial flutter can be converted to sinus rhythm with electrical cardioversion in the same way as for AF, although often with lower energy levels. Although drug therapy can be used to help maintain sinus rhythm in the long term, it is usually preferable to consider radiofrequency ablation of the atrial flutter circuit as it has a success rate >95%.

Great care has to be taken if flecainide is used in the treatment of paroxysmal atrial flutter. Flecainide can cause a paradoxical increase in ventricular rate (due to slowing of the atrial rate, which then facilitates 1:1 AV node conduction). If flecainide is used in the treatment of atrial flutter, it is usually given in conjunction with a negative chronotrope such as a beta blocker or digoxin to reduce the risk of high ventricular rates.

Atrial flutter carries a risk of thromboembolism, and patients with atrial flutter are usually assessed for antithrombotic therapy according to the same guidelines as those used in AF (see above).

## ATRIAL TACHYCARDIA

Atrial tachycardia differs from sinus tachycardia in that the impulses are generated by an ectopic focus somewhere within the atrial myocardium rather than the sinus node, as a result of increased automaticity, triggered activity or a re-entry circuit. Atrial tachycardia can be **focal** (arising from one small focus in the atria) or **multifocal** (arising from three or more foci), and can be paroxysmal or sustained. Atrial flutter (p. 64) is often considered as a subtype of atrial tachycardia.

The atrial (P wave) rate is usually 100–250/min, with abnormally shaped P waves (Fig. 7.11). Above atrial rates of 200/min, the AV node struggles to keep up with impulse conduction and AV block may occur. The combination of focal atrial

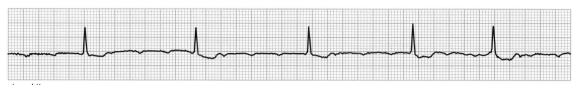

Lead II

**Figure 7.11** Atrial tachycardia.

Key points:
- There are inverted P waves (in lead II) indicating an atrial rhythm arising from near the AV node.
- The atrial rate is 167/min. There is variable AV block, so the ventricular rhythm is irregular and 40–60/min.

tachycardia with AV block is particularly common in digoxin toxicity. If the patient is not taking digoxin, consider:

- ischaemic heart disease
- chronic pulmonary disease
- rheumatic heart disease
- cardiomyopathy
- sick sinus syndrome (p. 57).

Non-sustained episodes of focal atrial tachycardia are commonly seen on ambulatory ECG monitoring, and are often asymptomatic. Sustained atrial tachycardia can lead to a tachycardia-induced cardiomyopathy, and it is particularly important not to misdiagnose the rhythm as sinus tachycardia in such cases.

Focal atrial tachycardia should be treated with urgent electrical cardioversion if the patient is haemodynamically unstable. Stable patients may cardiovert with adenosine (in adenosine-sensitive cases), or with beta blockers or non-dihydropyridine calcium channel blockers (verapamil or diltiazem). If digoxin toxicity is the cause of the atrial tachycardia, the digoxin should of course be stopped. Rate control and/or prophylaxis against recurrent paroxysms of atrial tachycardia can be attained using beta blockers or non-dihydropyridine calcium channel blockers. Catheter ablation is also a treatment option in such cases.

Multifocal atrial tachycardia can be mistaken for AF, due to its irregular nature, but closer inspection of the ECG will reveal P waves with at least three different morphologies. It is commonly associated with underlying chronic pulmonary disease or electrolyte abnormalities. Any contributory factors should be optimally treated, and long-term treatment is usually with calcium channel blockers (or beta blockers, if not contraindicated by pulmonary disease). There is no role for electrical cardioversion or catheter ablation.

## AV RE-ENTRY TACHYCARDIA

Conduction of impulses between the atria and the ventricles can normally only occur via one route, the AV node. However, some individuals have an additional connection between the atria and the ventricles, known as an **accessory pathway**. A left-sided accessory pathway, between the left atrium and left ventricle, is shown in Figure 7.12; however, accessory pathways can occur virtually anywhere in the annulus fibrosus, the fibrous ring separating the atria from the ventricles.

The presence of an accessory pathway means that there are *two* distinct routes for conduction of impulses between atria and ventricles – via the AV node, as normal,

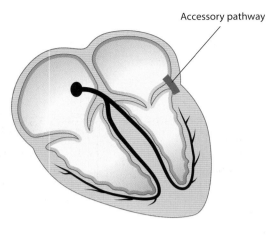

**Figure 7.12** Accessory pathway.

Key point:    • There is a left-sided accessory pathway, between the left atrium and the left ventricle.

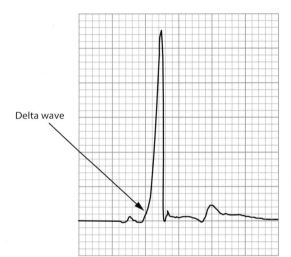

Delta wave

**Figure 7.13** Delta wave.

Key points:    • There is a slurred early upstroke to the QRS complex (a delta wave).
• Note that the PR interval is short.

and also via the accessory pathway. This provides a mechanism by which an AV re-entry tachycardia (AVRT) can occur. In AVRT, an impulse can travel down one route and back up the other, to form a continuous re-entry circuit.

Most accessory pathways can conduct impulses *antegradely* (from atria to ventricles). When antegrade conduction occurs during normal sinus rhythm, **ventricular pre-excitation** is evident on the ECG, in the form of a **delta wave** (a slurred early upstroke of the QRS complex, Fig. 7.13). In addition, because the accessory pathway conducts impulses very rapidly between atria and ventricles, lacking the intrinsic 'slowness' of the AV node, the **PR interval is short** (<0.12 s).

However, once the wave of depolarization reaches the ventricular myocardium via the accessory pathway, it then slows down because it hasn't got access to the normal His–Purkinje system. Instead, the impulse has to travel myocyte to myocyte, and because this is slower than normal the resulting QRS complex has a slow-rising 'slurred' initial upstroke. This is the delta wave of ventricular pre-excitation. Meanwhile, the wave of depolarization has *also* been travelling through the AV node, in the usual way, and when it reaches the His–Purkinje system the rest of the ventricular myocardium depolarizes rapidly (Fig. 7.14). Thus the slurred delta wave is followed by the rapid upstroke of an otherwise normal QRS complex.

When a short PR interval and delta wave are seen on an ECG, this is called a Wolff–Parkinson–White (WPW) *pattern*, and this is seen in approximately 0.2% of the general population (Fig. 7.15). The accessory pathway in individuals with

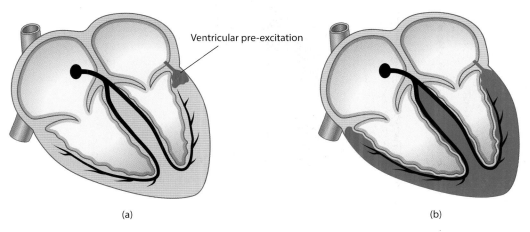

Ventricular pre-excitation

(a)  (b)

**Figure 7.14** Ventricular pre-excitation.

Key points:  (a) There is early activation of part of the ventricular myocardium via the accessory pathway.
(b) The remainder of the myocardium is depolarized in the normal way, via the AV node and the His–Purkinje system, shortly afterwards.

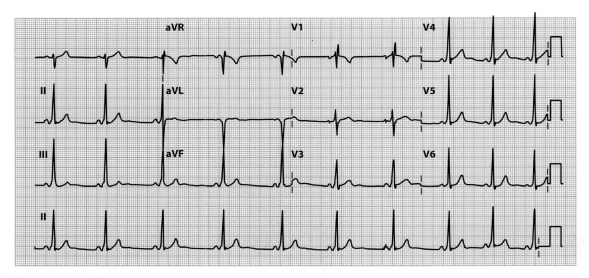

**Figure 7.15** Wolff–Parkinson–White pattern.

Key point:  • The PR interval is short, and there is a slurred early upstroke to the QRS complex (a delta wave).

a WPW pattern is known as the bundle of Kent. For most people with a WPW pattern on their ECG it is simply an incidental finding, and the presence of an accessory pathway never leads to any arrhythmias. However, for some, it acts as a substrate for AVRT, and these patients are then said to have WPW *syndrome*.

---

### SUBTYPES OF THE WPW ECG PATTERN

WPW ECG patterns are conventionally divided into two subtypes:

- Type A WPW pattern has a predominantly positive delta wave and QRS complex in the chest leads, with a positive R wave in lead $V_1$ which resembles a right bundle branch block pattern (Fig. 7.15). In type A, the accessory pathway lies on the left side of the heart.
- Type B WPW pattern has a predominantly negative delta wave and QRS complex in leads $V_1$–$V_2$, which resembles a left bundle branch block pattern. In type B, the accessory pathway lies on the right side of the heart.

---

Some patients with an accessory pathway have a normal ECG, with a normal PR interval and no delta wave – when an accessory pathway is not evident on the surface ECG, it is said to be a **concealed pathway**. In these cases, the accessory pathway is only capable of *retrograde* conduction, so the anterograde conduction that is responsible for ventricular pre-excitation cannot occur. However, these patients can still experience AVRT, during which the impulses travel down the AV node and back up the accessory pathway (orthodromic AVRT, see below).

## AVRT in WPW syndrome

In the vast majority (95%) of episodes of AVRT seen in patients with WPW syndrome, the re-entry circuit travels down the AV node and back up the accessory pathway (Fig. 7.16). This is known as an **orthodromic AVRT**, and is usually triggered by an atrial ectopic beat which occurs while the accessory pathway is refractory to conduction – this ectopic is therefore conducted down the AV node but not down the accessory pathway. However, by the time that the impulse subsequently reaches the ventricular side of the accessory pathway, the pathway is no longer refractory and can conduct the impulse retrogradely back up to the atria, thus setting up a re-entry circuit. The ECG during orthodromic AVRT (Fig. 7.17) shows:

- regular QRS complexes
- narrow QRS complexes
- heart rate 130–220/min.

An inverted P wave is often visible just after each QRS complex, representing retrograde activation of the atria each time the impulse re-enters the atria via the accessory pathway. Typically the interval between the R wave and the P wave is shorter than that between the P wave and the subsequent R wave – orthodromic AVRT is therefore known as a **short RP tachycardia**.

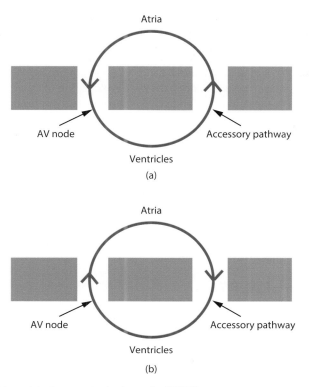

Figure 7.16 Atrioventricular re-entry tachycardia (AVRT).

Key points:     (a) Orthodromic AVRT.
                (b) Antidromic AVRT.

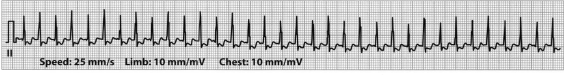

Lead II

Figure 7.17 Orthodromic atrioventricular re-entry tachycardia (AVRT).

Key point:     • There is a regular narrow-complex tachycardia (204/min) with inverted P waves (distorting the ST
                  segments) following each QRS complex.

Much less commonly, the re-entry circuit travels down the accessory pathway and back up through the AV node – this is an **antidromic AVRT**, and in this situation the QRS complexes are regular and *broad*. This occurs because the ventricles are depolarized via the accessory pathway, which means the impulses can't gain access to the His–Purkinje system and the depolarization has to occur from myocyte-to-myocyte (as with the delta wave, p. 129). The heart rate is typically faster, and symptoms more marked, in antidromic than in orthodromic AVRT. Antidromic AVRT can be very difficult to distinguish from ventricular tachycardia (VT), and indeed can act as a trigger for VT or for ventricular fibrillation (VF).

---

### ATRIAL FIBRILLATION IN WOLFF–PARKINSON–WHITE SYNDROME

AVRT is not the only arrhythmia that can occur in WPW syndrome. AF (or other atrial tachyarrhythmias, such as atrial flutter or atrial tachycardia) can occur, and are potentially life-threatening in this context. If a patient with an accessory pathway develops one of these atrial tachyarrhythmias, rapid conduction to the ventricles can occur via the accessory pathway, leading to a rapid ventricular rate and triggering ventricular tachycardia or fibrillation. Electrical cardioversion is the immediate treatment of choice if the patient is haemodynamically compromised. Patients with an accessory pathway who have had AF or other atrial tachyarrhythmias, or who are at high risk of doing so, should be urgently considered for catheter ablation of the pathway.

---

Symptoms of AVRT vary between patients. Palpitation is the commonest complaint but can vary greatly in duration and severity. Palpitation typically starts (and terminates) abruptly, and may be accompanied by chest pain, breathlessness, dizziness or syncope.

## Termination of AVRT

An episode of AVRT can be terminated by blocking the AV node, thereby breaking the re-entry circuit. The **Valsalva manoeuvre** increases vagal inhibition of AV nodal conduction, thus slowing AV nodal conduction and terminating the tachycardia. Alternatively, you can perform **carotid sinus massage** (while monitoring the ECG) with the same aim, as long as the patient does not have carotid bruits or any history of cerebrovascular events. The technique of carotid sinus massage is described on page 66.

---

### VALSALVA MANOEUVRE

The Valsalva manoeuvre describes the action of forced expiration against a closed glottis. To perform it, patients should be asked to breathe in and then to strain for a few seconds with their breath held. Alternatively, they can be given a 20-mL plastic syringe and asked to 'blow' into the hole to try to push out the plunger from the opposite end. This is impossible to achieve, but in trying to do so the patient effectively performs a Valsalva manoeuvre.

---

Drug treatments to terminate an episode of AVRT include intravenous adenosine (do not use if the patient has asthma or obstructive airways disease) or intravenous verapamil (not to be used if the patient has recently taken a beta blocker). If the patient is haemodynamically compromised, consider urgent electrical cardioversion (p. 63).

## Prevention of AVRT

In the longer term, AVRT may not require prophylactic treatment if episodes are brief and cause few symptoms. Patients can be taught to use the Valsalva manoeuvre. If longer-term drug treatment is required, options include sotalol, flecainide and propafenone. However, catheter ablation of the accessory pathway is curative in a very high proportion of cases, at relatively low risk, and so should be considered a first-line therapy in symptomatic patients with WPW syndrome.

AF, atrial flutter and atrial tachycardia carry considerable risk of sudden cardiac death in patients with an accessory pathway, and patients who have experienced these arrhythmias should be considered for urgent catheter ablation.

**SEEK HELP**

> Patients with an accessory pathway who have had symptomatic AVRT, or who have experienced AF, atrial flutter or atrial tachycardia, should be considered for a catheter ablation procedure. All patients with an accessory pathway, even if asymptomatic, should have an assessment by a cardiologist to determine their future risk of developing potentially hazardous arrhythmias.

## AV NODAL RE-ENTRY TACHYCARDIA

AVNRT is, like AVRT, a tachycardia that is based around a re-entry circuit. However, the re-entry circuit of AVNRT occurs on a much smaller scale than in AVRT, occurring in the tissues within or just adjacent to the AV node. This is sometimes referred to as a micro re-entry circuit (as opposed to the macro re-entry circuit in AVRT).

In many individuals the AV nodal tissue contains two distinct pathways – called fast and slow – and the normal conduction of sinus beats occurs via the fast pathway (Fig. 7.18). This is because, when a sinus beat reaches the AV node, it starts to be conducted simultaneously down both fast *and* slow pathways. Because it travels more quickly down the fast pathway, the impulse down the fast pathway arrives at the point where the fast and slow pathways meet before the impulse down the slow pathway does. The impulse that has travelled down the fast pathway then starts travelling retrogradely up the slow pathway, meeting the impulse which is still making its way down the slow pathway, and blocking it.

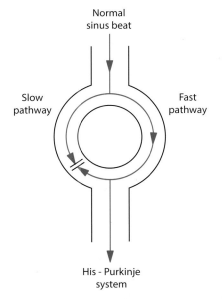

**Figure 7.18** Atrioventricular (AV) nodal conduction.

Key point:    • Normal AV nodal conduction occurs via the fast pathway.

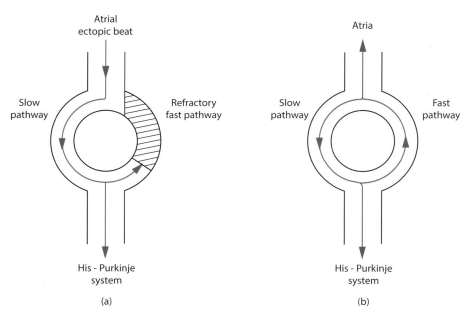

**Figure 7.19** Atrioventricular nodal re-entry tachycardia (AVNRT).

Key points:   (a) An atrial ectopic beat travels down the slow pathway when the fast pathway is refractory.
(b) The impulse then conducts back up the fast pathway, which has recovered from its refractory period.

However, if an atrial ectopic beat occurs at just the right moment, a re-entry circuit can be set up (Fig. 7.19). For this to happen, the atrial ectopic beat has to arrive while the fast pathway is refractory. The beat will therefore travel down the slow pathway, but by the time it reaches the point where the two pathways meet, the fast pathway has recovered from its refractory period. This means that the impulse can now travel up the fast pathway, and then back down the slow pathway, *ad infinitum*, leading to an AVNRT. This is known as the **slow-fast** (or typical) form of AVNRT, because antegrade conduction is via the slow pathway, and retrograde conduction via the fast pathway. The slow-fast form accounts for 90% of AVNRT cases seen.

With each circuit of the impulse, the atria and ventricles will be depolarized simultaneously. As a result, the (inverted) P waves are buried within the QRS complexes and can be difficult or impossible to discern. Like AVRT, typical slow-fast AVNRT is a **short RP tachycardia**, the interval between the R wave and the P wave being shorter than that between the P wave and the subsequent R wave. The ECG shows a regular narrow complex tachycardia, with a ventricular rate usually 180–250/min (Fig. 7.20).

Much less commonly, fast-slow (or atypical) AVNRT can occur, with antegrade conduction via the fast pathway and retrograde conduction via the slow pathway. There is also a slow-slow form of AVNRT, if more than one slow pathway is present. The inverted P waves are easier to see in these forms of AVNRT, as atrial depolarization occurs later than ventricular depolarization. These are **long RP tachycardias**,

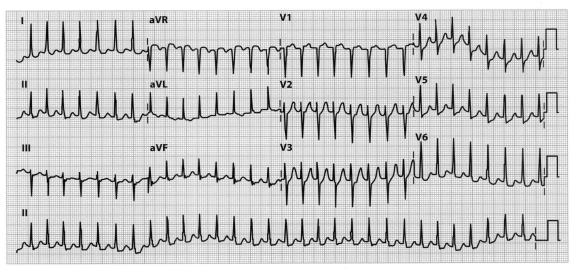

**Figure 7.20** Atrioventricular nodal re-entry tachycardia (AVNRT).

Key points:
- There is a regular narrow-complex tachycardia with a heart rate of 180/min.
- P waves can just be discerned at the end of the QRS complexes in some of the leads.

the interval between the R wave and the P wave being longer than that between the P wave and the subsequent R wave.

Distinguishing between AVNRT and AVRT can be difficult, although an ECG in sinus rhythm may help (as it may reveal evidence of ventricular pre-excitation, supporting a diagnosis of AVRT). The definitive diagnosis can prove challenging, however, and sometimes requires electrophysiological studies.

Symptoms of AVNRT vary greatly between patients. Palpitation is the commonest complaint but can vary in duration and severity. Palpitation tends to be of abrupt onset and termination, and may be accompanied by chest pain, breathlessness, dizziness or syncope.

## Treatment of AVNRT

As with AVRT (p. 67), an episode of AVNRT can be terminated by blocking the AV node, thereby breaking the cycle of electrical activity. This can be achieved using the **Valsalva manoeuvre** or with **carotid sinus massage** (while monitoring the ECG), as described earlier.

Drug treatments to terminate an episode of AVNRT include intravenous adenosine (do not use if the patient has asthma or obstructive airways disease) or intravenous verapamil (not to be used if the patient has recently taken a beta blocker). If the patient is haemodynamically compromised, consider urgent electrical cardioversion (although this is seldom necessary).

In the longer term, catheter ablation is the treatment of choice for symptomatic patients – the procedure performed involves ablation or modification of the slow pathway, which is effective in both typical and atypical forms of AVNRT (success rate 98%, with a recurrence rate <5%). Long-term drug therapy is often ineffective, but if patients prefer to avoid catheter ablation then drug options include verapamil, propranolol or digoxin.

**SEEK HELP**

Patients with AVNRT should be referred to a cardiologist for consideration of a catheter ablation procedure.

### SUPRAVENTRICULAR TACHYCARDIA

The term 'supraventricular tachycardia' is frequently misused and this leads to misunderstanding. Literally, it refers to any heart rate over 100/min (tachycardia) that originates above the ventricles (supraventricular). It encompasses many different arrhythmias, including sinus tachycardia, AF, atrial flutter, atrial tachycardia and AVRT/AVNRT. This is the meaning of SVT that has been used in this book. Some people use the term SVT to refer specifically to AVRT/AVNRT. However, we recommend that you identify all arrhythmias as specifically as possible, and reserve SVT as a general term for tachycardias that originate above the ventricles.

## SUMMARY

Supraventricular rhythms are those which arise above the level of the ventricles, i.e. from the sinoatrial (SA) node, the atria or the atrioventricular (AV) node. These include:

- sinus rhythm
- sinus arrhythmia
- sinus bradycardia
- sinus tachycardia
- sick sinus syndrome
- atrial ectopic beats
- atrial fibrillation
- atrial flutter
- atrial tachycardia
- focal atrial tachycardia
- multifocal atrial tachycardia
- atrioventricular re-entry tachycardia (AVRT)
- atrioventricular nodal re-entry tachycardia (AVNRT)

## FURTHER READING

Blomström-Lundqvist C, Scheinman MM, Aliot EM, *et al.* ACC/AHA/ESC guidelines for the management of patients with supraventricular arrhythmias – executive summary. *J Am Coll Cardiol* 2003; **42**: 1493–1531.

Camm AJ, Kirchhof P, Lip GY, *et al.* Guidelines for the management of atrial fibrillation: the Task Force for the Management of Atrial Fibrillation of the European Society of Cardiology (ESC). *Europace* 2010; **12**: 1360–1420.

Camm AJ, Lip GYH, De Caterina R, *et al.* 2012 focused update of the ESC guidelines for the management of atrial fibrillation. *Eur Heart J* 2012; **33**: 2719–2747.

Katritsis DG, Camm AJ. Atrioventricular nodal reentrant tachycardia. *Circulation* 2010; **122**: 831–840.

Whinnett ZI, Sohaib SMA, Davies DW. Diagnosis and management of supraventricular tachycardia. *BMJ* 2012; **345**: e7769.

# CHAPTER 8

# Ventricular rhythms

Ventricular rhythms are those which arise from the ventricles, i.e. below the level of the atrioventricular node. The ventricular rhythms we will consider are:

- ventricular ectopic beats
- accelerated idioventricular rhythm
- monomorphic ventricular tachycardia (VT)
- polymorphic ventricular tachycardia
- ventricular fibrillation (VF).

## VENTRICULAR ECTOPIC BEATS

Like atrial and AV junctional ectopic beats (p. 58), ventricular ectopic beats (VEBs) appear *earlier* than expected. VEBs are also called ventricular extrasystoles, ventricular premature complexes (VPCs), ventricular premature beats (VPBs) or premature ventricular contractions (PVCs).

VEBs are identified by a QRS complex that is broad and appears earlier than expected (Fig. 8.1). Because VEBs arise within the ventricular myocardium, the impulse cannot get a 'foothold' within the His-Purkinje conduction system. As a result, conduction of the impulse has to occur slowly from myocyte to myocyte, and so ventricular depolarization is slower than usual, which is why the QRS complex is broad (>0.12 s).

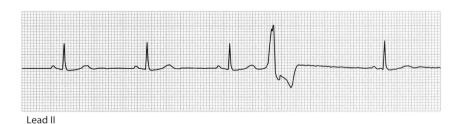

Lead II

**Figure 8.1** Ventricular ectopic beat.

Key point:  • After three normal sinus beats, there is a ventricular ectopic beat, followed by another normal sinus beat.

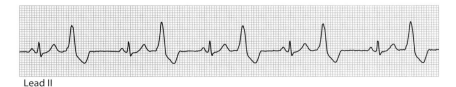

Lead II

**Figure 8.2** Ventricular bigeminy.

Key point:  • Every normal complex is followed by a ventricular ectopic beat.

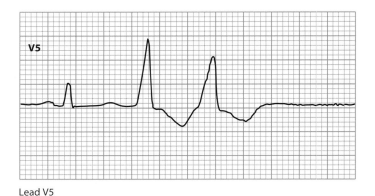

Lead V5

**Figure 8.3** Ventricular couplet.

Key point:    • Two ventricular ectopic beats occurring in succession are called a ventricular couplet.

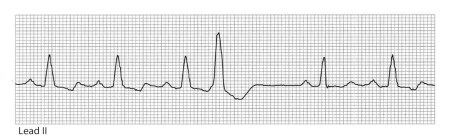

Lead II

**Figure 8.4** 'R on T' ventricular ectopic beat.

Key point:    • A ventricular ectopic beat occurs on the T wave of the third sinus beat.

Isolated VEBs are common, being seen in 40–75% of individuals during ambulatory ECG monitoring. VEBs may be asymptomatic, or may be experienced by the patient as a sensation of 'extra' and/or 'missed' heartbeats.

VEBs are usually called 'frequent' when they occur at a rate >60 per hour (although different definitions of 'frequent' are used by different authors). Multiple VEBs which share the same QRS complex morphology originate from a single focus within the ventricles and are therefore called **unifocal**. Where the VEBs have two or more different morphologies, they arise from different foci and are called **multifocal**.

There may be a regular pattern to the occurrence of VEBs: where every normal beat is followed by a VEB, the patient is said to be in **ventricular bigeminy** (Fig. 8.2). If every third beat is a VEB, this is **ventricular trigeminy**, and if every fourth beat is a VEB, this is **ventricular quadrigeminy**. A pair of VEBs occurring in succession is called a **ventricular couplet** (Fig. 8.3). Three or more VEBs in succession is **ventricular tachycardia** (p. 83).

Occasionally, VEBs will be followed by inverted P waves if the atria are activated by retrograde conduction via the AV node. If retrograde conduction does not occur, there will usually be a full compensatory pause before the next normal beat because the sinoatrial node will not be 'reset'. VEBs can occur at the same time as the T wave of the preceding beat – such 'R on T' VEBs (Fig. 8.4) can act as a trigger for ventricular arrhythmias.

There are many potential causes of VEBs, including:

- myocardial ischaemia/infarction
- electrolyte disturbance (e.g. hypokalaemia, hypomagnesaemia)
- myocarditis
- cardiomyopathy
- caffeine
- alcohol
- sympathomimetic drugs
- digoxin toxicity.

VEBs can be harmless, particularly when the heart is structurally normal, but can also be associated with more hazardous arrhythmias, especially when heart disease is present. Assessment of the patient with ventricular ectopics should therefore include a search for any underlying heart disease, which may include (in addition to a 12-lead ECG) echocardiography, ambulatory ECG monitoring and assessment for myocardial ischaemia.

The 12-lead ECG can be used as a guide to where VEBs originate from:

1. VEBs arising from the right ventricle will have a left bundle branch block (LBBB) morphology – this is because a right ventricular VEB will depolarize the right ventricle before the left, which is the same as the sequence of depolarization seen in LBBB.

2. Similarly, VEBs arising from the left ventricle will have a right bundle branch block (RBBB) morphology.

3. VEBs arising from the apex of the ventricles will have a superior axis, as demonstrated by negative (predominantly downward) QRS complexes in the inferior leads (II, III and aVF). This is because a VEB arising near the apex will depolarize the ventricles from apex to base, i.e. in a 'superior' direction, directed away from the inferior leads.

4. VEBs arising from the base of the ventricles will have an inferior axis, as demonstrated by positive (predominantly upright) QRS complexes in the inferior leads. This is because a VEB arising near the base will depolarize the ventricles from base to apex, i.e. in an 'inferior' direction, directed towards the inferior leads.

These principles are summarized in Table 8.1. It is therefore relatively simple to work out roughly where a VEB has arisen from, so long as it is captured in the appropriate leads on a 12-lead ECG (Fig. 8.5).

Commonly, VEBs are found to arise from the right ventricular base, usually from the right ventricular outflow tract (RVOT). Although RVOT VEBs can be associated with non-sustained VT ('RVOT VT'), they have traditionally been regarded

**Table 8.1** How to determine the origin of ventricular ectopic beats (VEBs)

| | | VEB morphology | |
| --- | --- | --- | --- |
| | | LBBB | RBBB |
| VEB axis | Inferior (positive QRS in inferior leads) | Right ventricle (base) | Left ventricle (base) |
| | Superior (negative QRS in inferior leads) | Right ventricle (apex) | Left ventricle (apex) |

8 Ventricular rhythms

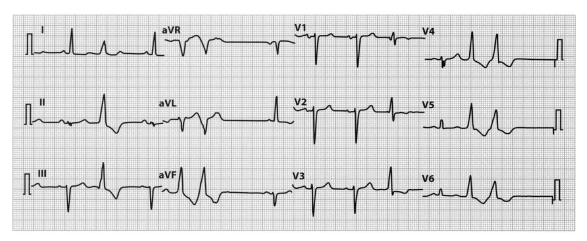

**Figure 8.5** Ventricular ectopic beats arising from the right ventricular base (right ventricular outflow tract).

Key points:
- Several ventricular ectopic beats/couplets are visible, with a left bundle branch block morphology (right ventricular origin) and an inferior axis (positive QRS in inferior leads).
- This indicates an origin at the right ventricular base, commonly in the right ventricular outflow tract.

as being associated with a generally good prognosis (although this assumption has been challenged, and many cases have been reported in which malignant ventricular arrhythmias have occurred). So-called 'benign' RVOT VEBs should not be confused with the similar VEBs that are seen in arrhythmogenic right ventricular cardiomyopathy, which carries a much more sinister prognosis. Careful imaging of the right ventricle with echocardiography and/or cardiac magnetic resonance imaging is therefore important to distinguish between these conditions in patients with VEBs arising from the right ventricle.

Even though some VEBs can precipitate fatal arrhythmias, routine treatment of incidental VEBs with anti-arrhythmic drugs has *not* been shown to decrease mortality. Some patients may be considerably troubled by symptoms caused by the VEBs and will benefit from using an anti-arrhythmic agent, as may patients who have experienced a potentially dangerous arrhythmia. Where feasible, catheter ablation can be considered where symptoms are troublesome or there is a risk of malignant arrhythmias, and an implantable cardioverter-defibrillator (ICD) is also an option to provide protection from dangerous arrhythmias.

## ACCELERATED IDIOVENTRICULAR RHYTHM

Accelerated idioventricular rhythm is essentially a slow form of VT, with a heart rate of less than 120 beats/min (Fig. 8.6). It occurs when an ectopic focus within the ventricles starts firing with a rate just higher than that of the sinoatrial node – this ventricular focus then takes over the cardiac rhythm.

Accelerated idioventricular rhythm is usually well tolerated and essentially 'benign' – it is not usually necessary to treat it with anti-arrhythmic drugs (indeed, trying to suppress accelerated idioventricular rhythm can lead to disastrous decompensation).

It is most commonly seen in the context of myocardial reperfusion during the treatment of an acute myocardial infarction. Other causes include electrolyte

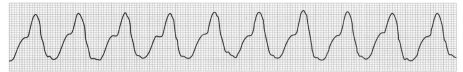

Lead II

**Figure 8.6** Accelerated idioventricular rhythm.

Key point:     • There is a broad complex (ventricular) rhythm with a rate of 88 beats/min.

abnormalities (which may require correction), myocarditis, cardiomyopathy and following cardiac arrest.

## MONOMORPHIC VENTRICULAR TACHYCARDIA

VT is a **broad-complex tachycardia**, defined as three or more successive ventricular beats at a heart rate above 100 beats/min and with a QRS complex duration >0.12 s (Fig. 8.7). VT arises most commonly as a re-entry circuit around an area of myocardial scarring (for instance, as a result of myocardial infarction). Other less common mechanisms include increased automaticity of a specific ventricular focus and abnormal triggering. Common clinical causes of VT are listed in Table 8.2.

An episode of VT can be described as:

- non-sustained (self-terminating in <30 s)
- sustained (lasting >30 s, or requiring urgent termination within 30 s due to haemodynamic compromise)

and also as:

- monomorphic (arising from a single ventricular focus, with a uniform QRS complex morphology)
- polymorphic (with a changing focus and thus a varying QRS complex morphology).

Polymorphic VT is discussed in more detail on page 89.

Sustained VT usually occurs at a heart rate of 150–250/min, but this can be well tolerated and may not cause haemodynamic disturbance. Do *not* assume, therefore, that just because the patient appears well, they do not have VT. The symptoms of VT can vary from mild palpitations to dizziness, syncope and cardiac arrest.

Choose the urgency and the type of treatment required according to the clinical state of the patient. When a patient has pulseless VT, they are in cardiac arrest and should be managed in accordance with the Adult Advanced Life Support algorithm (Fig. 8.8). Where a patient with VT has a pulse, they should be managed in line with the Adult Tachycardia (With Pulse) algorithm (Fig. 5.5).

**ACT QUICKLY**

Ventricular tachycardia is a medical emergency. Urgent diagnosis and treatment are required.

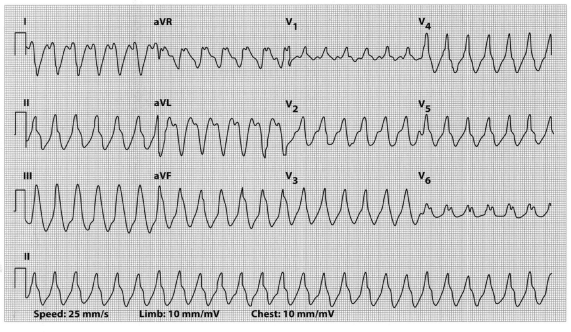

**Figure 8.7** Ventricular tachycardia.

Key points:   • There is a broad complex tachycardia with a rate of 152 beats/min.
              • The QRS complex duration is 0.164 s.

**Table 8.2** Causes of ventricular tachycardia

- Myocardial ischaemia and infarction
- Dilated cardiomyopathy
- Hypertrophic cardiomyopathy
- Arrhythmogenic right ventricular cardiomyopathy
- Myocarditis
- Congenital heart disease (repaired or unrepaired)
- Electrolyte disturbances
- Pro-arrhythmic drugs
- Right ventricular outflow tract tachycardia
- Long QT syndrome
- Brugada syndrome

Following the initial management and correction of VT, longer-term management should be discussed with a cardiologist. Long-term prophylaxis is usually not necessary for VT occurring within the first 48 h following an acute myocardial infarction. Where prophylaxis is needed, effective drug treatments include sotalol (particularly when VT is exercise related) or amiodarone. Ventricular tachycardia related to bradycardia should be treated by pacing. Ablation or surgery can be used to remove a ventricular focus or re-entry circuit identified by electrophysiological testing. Finally, ICDs can be implanted to deliver overdrive pacing and/or shocks for recurrent episodes of VT and VF (Chapter 20).

8 Ventricular rhythms

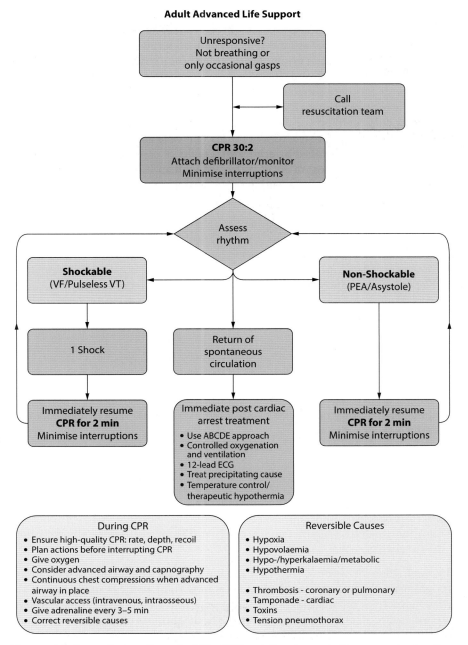

**Adult Advanced Life Support**

Unresponsive?
Not breathing or
only occasional gasps

Call
resuscitation team

**CPR 30:2**
Attach defibrillator/monitor
Minimise interruptions

Assess
rhythm

**Shockable**
(VF/Pulseless VT)

**Non-Shockable**
(PEA/Asystole)

1 Shock

Return of
spontaneous
circulation

Immediately resume
**CPR for 2 min**
Minimise interruptions

Immediate post cardiac
arrest treatment
• Use ABCDE approach
• Controlled oxygenation
  and ventilation
• 12-lead ECG
• Treat precipitating cause
• Temperature control/
  therapeutic hypothermia

Immediately resume
**CPR for 2 min**
Minimise interruptions

**During CPR**
• Ensure high-quality CPR: rate, depth, recoil
• Plan actions before interrupting CPR
• Give oxygen
• Consider advanced airway and capnography
• Continuous chest compressions when advanced
  airway in place
• Vascular access (intravenous, intraosseous)
• Give adrenaline every 3–5 min
• Correct reversible causes

**Reversible Causes**
• Hypoxia
• Hypovolaemia
• Hypo-/hyperkalaemia/metabolic
• Hypothermia

• Thrombosis - coronary or pulmonary
• Tamponade - cardiac
• Toxins
• Tension pneumothorax

**Figure 8.8** Resuscitation Council (UK) 2010 adult advanced life support algorithm. ABCDE – Airway, Breathing, Circulation, Disability, Exposure (see p. 46); CPR – cardiopulmonary resuscitation; PEA – pulseless electrical activity; VF – ventricular fibrillation; VT – ventricular tachycardia. Reproduced with the kind permission of the Resuscitation Council (UK).

8 Ventricular rhythms

VT can be idiopathic in the context of an apparently structurally normal heart – in this context, the most common type is right ventricular outflow tract (RVOT) tachycardia, which accounts for around 10 per cent of all forms of VT. It is often seen in association with ventricular ectopic beats, which have a characteristic appearance of left bundle branch block and an inferior axis indicative of their RVOT origin. The prognosis for these patients is generally good. It is important, however, not to mistake the relatively benign RVOT form of VT with VT caused by arrhythmogenic right ventricular cardiomyopathy (ARVC), which has a more sinister prognosis. In ARVC the heart is *not* structurally normal, and the abnormal right ventricular morphology can be identified by echocardiography or cardiac magnetic resonance imaging. VT in the context of ARVC is treated with an ICD, whereas symptomatic RVOT tachycardia is usually treated with ablation.

---

### BRUGADA SYNDROME

Be careful not to miss Brugada syndrome in patients presenting with ventricular arrhythmias, including VT and VF. The heart appears structurally normal in this condition, but the presence of an abnormality of the cardiac sodium channel predisposes to potentially lethal arrhythmias. Brugada syndrome is characterized on the ECG by a right bundle branch block morphology and persistent ST segment elevation in leads $V_1$–$V_3$. The condition is discussed in more detail on page 170.

---

**SEEK HELP**

Patients who have experienced VT may benefit from implantation of an ICD. Their management options should be discussed with a cardiologist.

## HOW DO I DISTINGUISH BETWEEN VT AND SVT?

VT causes a broad complex tachycardia on the ECG. However, a broad complex tachycardia can also result from a supraventricular tachycardia (SVT) with aberrant conduction (such as a bundle branch block, p. 153, or ventricular pre-excitation, p. 68; see also Table 8.3).

The distinction between VT and SVT with aberrant conduction is not always straightforward. However, the distinction is important as the management of the two conditions is different (although in an emergency both VT and SVT usually respond to electrical cardioversion). When the diagnosis is unclear, the overriding principle is that **broad-complex tachycardia is always assumed to be VT unless proven otherwise.**

**Table 8.3** Broad-complex vs narrow-complex rhythms

|  | Broad complex | Narrow complex |
| --- | :---: | :---: |
| Supraventricular rhythm with normal conduction | X | ✓ |
| Supraventricular rhythm with aberrant conduction | ✓ | X |
| Ventricular rhythm | ✓ | X |

Most cases (80%) of broad complex tachycardia are due to VT, and the likelihood of VT (rather than SVT with aberrant conduction) is even higher when structural heart disease is present. Haemodynamic stability is not a reliable guide in distinguishing between VT and SVT with aberrant conduction, as VT can be remarkably well tolerated by some patients.

A very reliable ECG indicator of VT is the presence of **atrioventricular dissociation**, where the atria and ventricles are seen to be working independently. Unfortunately, such features are seen in fewer than half of cases of VT, so the absence of independent atrial activity doesn't exclude VT as a diagnosis. Atrioventricular dissociation is indicated by:

- independent P wave activity
- fusion beats
- capture beats.

**Independent P wave activity** is shown by the presence of P waves occurring at a slower rate than the QRS complexes and bearing no relation to them (Fig. 8.9).

**Fusion beats** appear when the ventricles are activated by an atrial impulse and a ventricular impulse arriving simultaneously (Fig. 8.10).

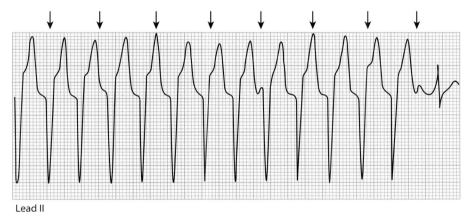

Lead II

**Figure 8.9** Independent P wave activity.

Key points:
- There is a broad-complex tachycardia (VT).
- The arrows show independent P waves deforming the QRS complexes.
- The last beat is a capture beat.

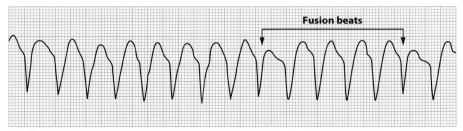

Lead II

**Figure 8.10** Fusion beats.

Key points:
- There is a broad-complex tachycardia (VT).
- The arrows show fusion beats.

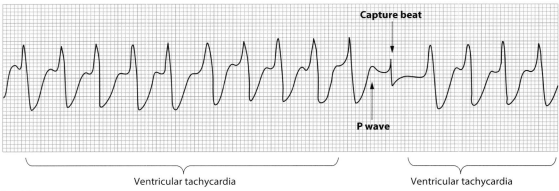

**Figure 8.11** Capture beats.

Key points:    • There is a broad-complex tachycardia (VT).
              • There is one normal QRS complex (capture beat).

**Capture beats** occur when an atrial impulse manages to 'capture' the ventricles for a beat, causing a normal QRS complex, which may be preceded by a normal P wave (Fig. 8.11).

Other ECG features can also provide clues to the diagnosis. Most patients with SVT and aberrant conduction will have a QRS complex morphology that looks like a typical LBBB or RBBB pattern. Patients with VT will often (but not always) have more unusual-looking QRS complexes which don't fit a typical bundle branch block pattern.

Many other ECG features suggest (but do not prove) a diagnosis of VT rather than SVT with aberrant conduction, including:

- very broad QRS complexes (>160 ms)
- extreme QRS axis deviation (p. 118)
- concordance (same QRS direction) in leads $V_1$–$V_6$
- an interval >100 ms from the start of the R wave to the deepest point of the S wave (this is called Brugada's sign) in one chest lead
- a notch in the downstroke of the S wave (this is called Josephson's sign).

Some of these features are formalized into a stepwise approach known as the **Brugada algorithm**:

**Step 1** – Is the RS complex absent across all the chest leads? If yes, then the diagnosis is VT; if no, move on to:

**Step 2** – Is the R to S interval >100 ms in one chest lead? If yes, then the diagnosis is VT; if no, move on to:

**Step 3** – Is atrioventricular dissociation present? If yes, then the diagnosis is VT; if no, move on to:

**Step 4** – Assess leads $V_1$–$V_2$ and lead $V_6$ for morphological criteria for VT:

- In the presence of an RBBB pattern, VT is suggested by:
  - monophasic R wave in lead $V_1$
  - R larger than R' in lead $V_1$
  - S greater than R in lead $V_6$

- In the presence of an LBBB pattern, VT is suggested by:
  - broad R wave (>30 ms) in lead $V_1$ or $V_2$
  - interval >60 ms to the deepest point of the S wave in lead $V_1$ or $V_2$
  - Q wave in lead $V_6$.

The termination of a broad complex tachycardia by a manoeuvre to block the atrioventricular node (such as a Valsalva manoeuvre, carotid sinus massage or the administration of intravenous adenosine) is highly suggestive of supraventricular tachycardia with aberrant conduction. However, some rare forms of VT can also respond to adenosine (and also to verapamil), the commonest of which is fascicular VT arising from the posterior fascicle of the left bundle branch.

## POLYMORPHIC VENTRICULAR TACHYCARDIA

In contrast to monomorphic VT, polymorphic VT is distinguished by a *varying* QRS complex morphology (Fig. 8.12). Like monomorphic VT, polymorphic VT can be classified as sustained or non-sustained. Polymorphic VT falls into two distinct categories based upon the duration of the QT interval (measured during sinus rhythm):

- polymorphic VT in the setting of a normal QT interval
- polymorphic VT in the setting of a prolonged QT interval.

When the underlying QT interval is normal, polymorphic VT may be due to myocardial ischaemia/infarction, coronary reperfusion (following myocardial infarction), structural heart disease or the rare condition of catecholaminergic polymorphic VT.

When polymorphic VT is seen in the context of a prolonged QT interval, it is commonly called **torsades de pointes** ('twisting of the points'). There are several causes of QT interval prolongation, including hypocalcaemia, acute myocarditis, long QT syndrome and certain drugs. QT interval prolongation, and its management, are discussed further on page 192.

Polymorphic VT carries a risk of precipitating VF and so urgent assessment (with involvement of a cardiologist) is warranted. In an emergency, standard adult life support protocols (Figs. 5.5 and 8.8) should be followed including urgent defibrillation if required. Treat underlying causes, such as myocardial ischaemia/infarction or electrolyte abnormalities, and stop any causative drugs. If the underlying QT interval is prolonged, useful measures can also include the administration of

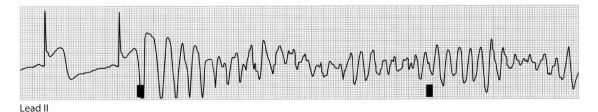

Lead II

**Figure 8.12** Polymorphic ventricular tachycardia.

Key points:
- This patient presented with an inferior ST-segment elevation myocardial infarction.
- An R on T ventricular ectopic beat triggers ventricular tachycardia with a continuously varying QRS complex morphology.

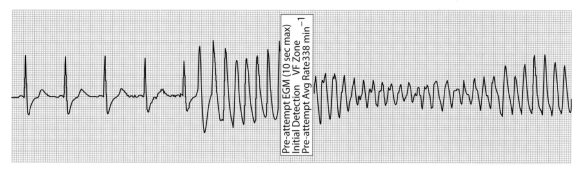

Pre-attempt EGM (10 sec max)    VF Zone
Initial Detection
Pre-attempt Avg Rate338 min⁻¹

**Figure 8.13** Polymorphic ventricular tachycardia.

Key point:    • This episode of polymorphic ventricular tachycardia was detected by an implantable cardioverter-defibrillator, prior to the device delivering a shock to correct the rhythm.

intravenous magnesium and consideration of temporary transvenous pacing (which increases the heart rate and thereby shortens the QT interval). In the longer term, an ICD may be required if the patient is judged to be at high risk of recurrent arrhythmias and sudden cardiac death. Figure 8.13 shows an ECG recording downloaded from an ICD following an episode of polymorphic VT.

**SEEK HELP**

Polymorphic VT can cause sudden cardiac death. Urgent involvement of a cardiologist is recommended.

## VENTRICULAR FIBRILLATION

In VF the ECG shows a chaotic rhythm without clearly discernible P waves, QRS complexes or T waves (Fig. 8.14). VF is sometimes called 'coarse' or 'fine' depending upon the amplitude of the chaotic activity on the ECG. Untreated VF is a rapidly fatal arrhythmia. It therefore requires immediate diagnosis and treatment according to the Adult Advanced Life Support algorithm (Fig. 8.8).

Ventricular fibrillation can occur in the context of:

- myocardial ischaemia/infarction
- cardiomyopathy
- myocarditis
- electrolyte disturbances
- pro-arrhythmic drugs
- long QT syndrome
- Brugada syndrome
- cardiac trauma
- electrical shock.

Always check for reversible causes following an episode of VF. In the longer term, an ICD (Chapter 20) should be considered for survivors of VF who are considered to be

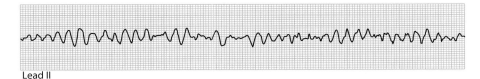

Lead II

**Figure 8.14** Ventricular fibrillation.

Key point:    • This rhythm strip demonstrates the chaotic rhythm of ventricular fibrillation.

at risk of recurrent VF. Such patients may also require appropriate anti-arrhythmic medication (e.g. amiodarone, beta blockers) to reduce the risk of recurrence.

 **ACT QUICKLY**

Ventricular fibrillation is a medical emergency. Immediate diagnosis and treatment are essential.

## SUMMARY

Ventricular rhythms are those which arise from the ventricles, i.e. below the level of the atrioventricular node. These include:

- ventricular ectopic beats
- accelerated idioventricular rhythm
- monomorphic ventricular tachycardia (VT)
- polymorphic ventricular tachycardia
- ventricular fibrillation (VF).

## FURTHER READING

Alzand BSN, Crijns HJGM. Diagnostic criteria of broad QRS complex tachycardia: decades of evolution. *Europace* 2011; **13**: 465–472.

Brugada P, Brugada J, Mont L, *et al*. A new approach to the differential diagnosis of a regular tachycardia with a wide QRS complex. *Circulation* 1991; **83**: 1649–1659.

Jastrzebski M, Kukla P, Czarnecka D, *et al*. Comparison of five electrocardiographic methods for differentiation of wide QRS-complex tachycardias. *Europace* 2012; **14**: 1165–1171.

Ng GA. Treating patients with ventricular ectopic beats. *Heart* 2006; **92**; 1707–1712.

NICE Guideline TA95 – Implantable cardioverter defibrillators. Available for download from: http://guidance.nice.org.uk/TA95

Vereckei A, Duray G, Szénási G, *et al*. Application of a new algorithm in the differential diagnosis of wide QRS complex tachycardia. *Eur Heart J* 2007; **28**: 589–600.

8 Ventricular rhythms

# CHAPTER 9

# Conduction problems

As we discussed in Chapter 6, there are two questions to ask in assessing the cardiac rhythm:

- Where does the impulse arise from?
- How is the impulse conducted?

In Chapters 7 and 8 we looked at how different supraventricular and ventricular rhythms arise. In this chapter, we will look at how problems can occur with the subsequent conduction of these rhythms.

The normal conduction of impulses from the sinoatrial (SA) node to the ventricles was described in Chapter 1 – an impulse arises with spontaneous depolarization of the SA node, which then depolarizes the atria before reaching the atrioventricular (AV) node. The impulse then passes via the bundle of His to reach the left and right bundle branches, before depolarizing the ventricular myocardium via the Purkinje fibres.

Problems with conduction can occur at four key points in this pathway (Fig. 9.1):

- SA node
- AV node or bundle of His
- left or right bundle branches
- left anterior or posterior fascicles.

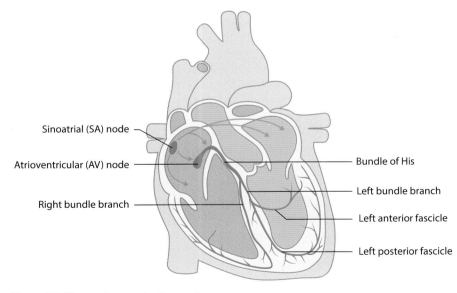

**Figure 9.1** The cardiac conduction system.

Key point: • Conduction block can occur at any of the points labelled.

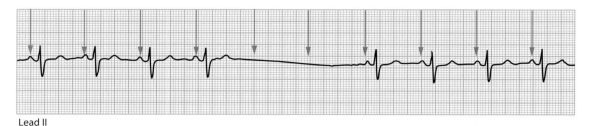

Lead II

**Figure 9.2** SA block.

Key points:
- The P waves are marked by arrows. There are two missing P waves as a result of SA block, but the next P wave appears exactly where you would predict.
- The SA node has therefore continued to depolarize, maintaining its cycle, but two of its impulses were blocked from depolarizing the atria.

## CONDUCTION BLOCK AT THE SA NODE

### SA block

If impulses are blocked from exiting the SA node, SA block (or SA 'exit' block) is said to occur. Because the impulse cannot leave the SA node, the atria do not depolarize and therefore a P wave is missing.

SA block is different to sinus arrest. In sinus arrest, the SA node does not depolarize at all; in SA block, the SA node *does* depolarize, but the impulse does not reach the rest of the atria. Both conditions lead to one or more missing P waves. However, in SA block the intrinsic rhythm of the SA node is maintained, so when the SA block resolves and a P wave finally does appear, it appears in the expected place (Fig. 9.2). In contrast, in sinus arrest the SA nodal rhythm is reset, and so the reappearance of the P wave is unpredictable.

## CONDUCTION BLOCK AT THE AV NODE OR BUNDLE OF HIS

When there are conduction problems at the AV node or bundle of His, conduction of impulses between the atria and ventricles is affected. This can take several forms or 'degrees'.

### First-degree AV block

In first-degree AV block, conduction through the AV node is slower than usual and the PR interval is therefore prolonged. Nonetheless, every P wave is followed by a QRS complex and therefore there are no 'dropped' beats.

The normal PR interval is 0.12–0.20 s, and so first-degree AV block is diagnosed when the PR interval measures >0.20 s (Fig. 9.3). The causes and treatment of first-degree AV block are discussed on page 130.

### Second-degree AV block

In second-degree AV block, there starts to be an intermittent failure of AV conduction and as a result some P waves are not followed by QRS complexes. There are three types of second-degree AV block:

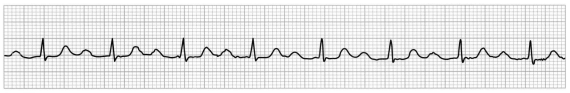

Lead II

**Figure 9.3** First-degree AV block.

Key point:    • The PR interval is prolonged at 0.28 s.

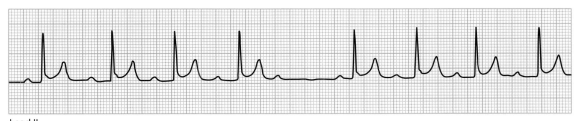

Lead II

**Figure 9.4** Mobitz type I AV block (Wenckebach phenomenon).

Key points:   • The PR interval gradually lengthens until a P wave fails to be conducted.
              • The PR interval resets, and the cycle repeats.

- if the PR interval gradually lengthens with each beat, until one P wave fails to produce a QRS complex, the patient has **Mobitz type I AV block**
- if the PR interval is fixed and normal, but occasionally a P wave fails to produce a QRS complex, the patient has **Mobitz type II AV block**
- if alternate P waves are not followed by QRS complexes, the patient has **2:1 AV block**.

**Mobitz type I AV block** (Fig. 9.4), also known as Wenckebach phenomenon, is usually a consequence of conduction problems within the AV node itself, sometimes simply as a result of high vagal tone – for instance, it is more commonly seen during sleep, and has a higher prevalence in athletes.

One can imagine Mobitz type I AV block as the AV node becoming increasingly 'tired' as it conducts each P wave – as a result, the node takes longer and longer to conduct each subsequent P wave until it totally 'gives up' and fails to conduct a P wave at all. This, however, gives the AV node a chance to 'rest', and by the time the next P wave arrives it is ready to conduct normally, before the cycle repeats itself.

Less frequently, Mobitz type I AV block results from conduction problems distal to the AV node (infranodal), in which case the QRS complexes may be wide and the outlook is less benign.

**Mobitz type II AV block** (Fig. 9.5) is usually a consequence of conduction problems distal to the AV node (infranodal). As a result, there is a higher risk of progression to third-degree AV block and the prognosis is therefore worse than for Mobitz type I AV block.

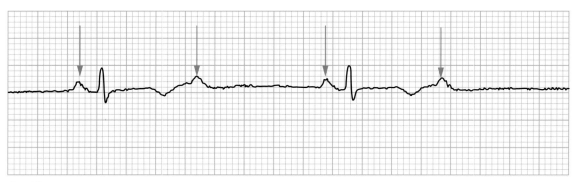

Lead II

**Figure 9.5** 2:1 AV block.

Key point:    • The P waves are marked by arrows. Only every alternate P wave is followed by a QRS complex.

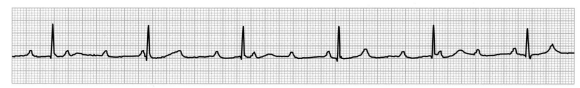

Lead II

**Figure 9.6** Third-degree AV block.

Key point:    • There is a complete block of AV conduction, with sinus rhythm in the atria and a narrow complex ('junctional') escape rhythm in the ventricles.

**2:1 AV block** is a form of second-degree AV block that cannot be categorized as Mobitz type I or type II. Because every alternate P wave is missing, it's impossible to say whether the PR interval would have lengthened or not. It's therefore traditional to consider 2:1 AV block as a category of second-degree heart block in its own right.

The management of each of these subtypes of second-degree AV block is discussed in Chapter 12.

### Third-degree AV block

In third-degree AV block ('complete heart block'), there is complete interruption of conduction between atria and ventricles, so that the two are working independently (Fig. 9.6). QRS complexes usually arise as the result of a ventricular escape rhythm (p. 102), in which the QRS complexes are usually broad. However, if the level of AV block is located in or just below the AV node, a junctional escape rhythm may arise with narrow QRS complexes.

Third-degree AV block can be congenital or acquired. In congenital cases, which are uncommon, the block is usually at the level of the AV node and is often associated with maternal anti-Ro or anti-La antibodies. Acquired cases can result from disease processes affecting the AV node and/or the infranodal conduction system (Table 9.1). The management of third-degree AV block is discussed page 133.

**Table 9.1** Causes of third-degree AV block

- Congenital
- Acquired
    - drug toxicity (e.g. anti-arrhythmics)
    - fibrosis/calcification of the conduction system
    - myocardial ischaemia/infarction
    - infection (e.g. Lyme disease)
    - myocardial infiltration (e.g. amyloid, sarcoid)
    - neuromuscular diseases (e.g. myotonic muscular dystrophy)
    - metabolic disorders (e.g. hypothyroidism)
    - cardiac procedures (e.g. ablation procedures, aortic valve surgery).

> **LYME DISEASE**
>
> In a patient with a recent onset of third-degree AV block, always consider the possibility of Lyme disease. This is transmitted by the spirochaete *Borrelia burgdorferi* and, in the second stage of the illness, can lead to first-degree, second-degree or third-degree AV block. The AV block can resolve entirely in response to antibiotics, although the patient may require support with a temporary pacemaker during treatment.

## CONDUCTION BLOCK AT THE BUNDLE BRANCHES

Moving down the conducting system beyond the bundle of His, **bundle branch block** can affect either the left or right bundle branch (Fig. 9.1). If both the left *and* right bundle branches are blocked, this is equivalent to third-degree AV block, as no impulses will reach the ventricular myocardium from the atria.

### Left bundle branch block

In left bundle branch block (LBBB) conduction down the left bundle has failed, and so the left ventricle cannot be depolarized in the normal way via its Purkinje fibres. However, the right ventricle can still depolarize normally via the still-functioning right bundle. The right ventricle therefore depolarizes first (and does so in its normal rapid way via its Purkinje fibres), but then this wave of depolarization spreads slowly across to the left ventricle, going from myocyte to myocyte, until the left ventricle has also depolarized.

This delay in left ventricular activation causes **interventricular dyssynchrony**, with the right ventricle depolarizing (and contracting) before the left ventricle, which has a deleterious effect on left ventricular function.

The ECG in LBBB has an appearance as shown in Fig. 9.7, with broad QRS complexes (due to the prolonged process of depolarization) and characteristic morphologies to the QRS complexes. In LBBB, the interventricular septum has to depolarize from right to left, a reversal of the normal pattern. This causes a small Q wave in lead $V_1$ and a small R wave in lead $V_6$ (Fig. 9.8). The right ventricle is depolarized normally via the right bundle branch, causing an R wave in lead $V_1$ and an S wave in lead $V_6$ (Fig. 9.9). Then, the left ventricle is depolarized by the right, causing an S wave in lead $V_1$ and another R wave (called R') in lead $V_6$ (Fig. 9.10).

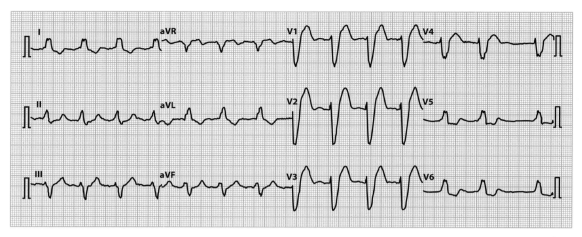

**Figure 9.7** Left bundle branch block.

Key points:  • There are broad QRS complexes, with a QRS complex morphology as explained in text.
           • The underlying rhythm in this case happens to be atrial fibrillation.

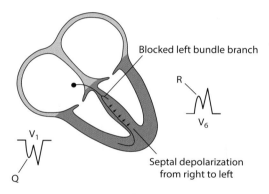

**Figure 9.8** Left bundle branch block – step one.

Key point:  • Septal depolarization occurs from right to left, leading to a small Q wave in lead $V_1$ and a small R wave in lead $V_6$.

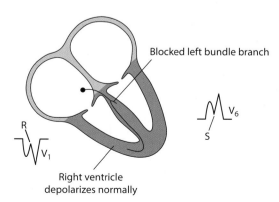

**Figure 9.9** Left bundle branch block – step two.

Key point:  • The right ventricle depolarizes normally, leading to an R wave in lead $V_1$ and an S wave in lead $V_6$.

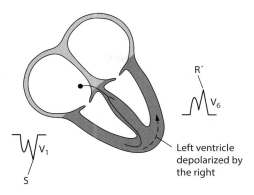

**Figure 9.10** Left bundle branch block – step three.

Key point:  • The left ventricle depolarizes late (via the right ventricle), leading to an S wave in lead $V_1$ and an R′ wave in lead $V_6$.

**Table 9.2** Causes of left bundle branch block

- Ischaemic heart disease
- Cardiomyopathy
- Left ventricular hypertrophy
- Hypertension
- Aortic stenosis
- Fibrosis of the conduction system

The presence of LBBB is almost invariably an indication of underlying pathology (Table 9.2), and the patient should be assessed accordingly. LBBB is discussed further in Chapter 14 (p. 153).

## Right bundle branch block

In contrast with LBBB, right bundle branch block (RBBB) is a relatively common finding in otherwise normal hearts. However, it too can result from underlying disease (Table 9.3) and should be investigated according to the clinical presentation.

In RBBB conduction down the right bundle has failed, and so the right ventricle cannot be depolarized in the normal way via its Purkinje fibres. However, the left ventricle can still depolarize normally via the still-functioning left bundle. The left ventricle therefore depolarizes first (and does so in its normal rapid way via its Purkinje fibres), but then this wave of depolarization spreads slowly across to the right ventricle, going from myocyte to myocyte, until the right ventricle has also depolarized. As with LBBB, this delay in right ventricular activation causes interventricular dyssynchrony.

**Table 9.3** Causes of right bundle branch block

- Ischaemic heart disease
- Cardiomyopathy
- Atrial septal defect
- Ebstein's anomaly
- Pulmonary embolism (usually massive)

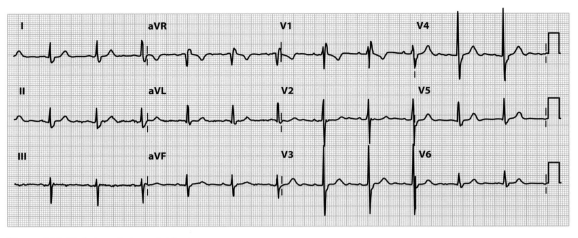

**Figure 9.11** Right bundle branch block.

Key point:    • There are broad QRS complexes, with a QRS complex morphology as explained in the text.

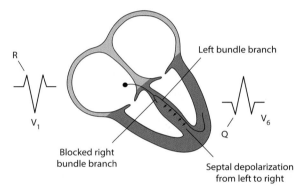

**Figure 9.12** Right bundle branch block – step one.

Key point:    • Septal depolarization occurs from left to right, leading to a small R wave in lead $V_1$ and a small 'septal' Q wave in lead $V_6$.

The ECG in RBBB has an appearance as shown in Fig. 9.11, with broad QRS complexes (due to the prolonged process of depolarization) and characteristic morphologies to the QRS complexes. In RBBB, the interventricular septum depolarizes normally, from left to right, causing a tiny R wave in lead $V_1$ and a small 'septal' Q wave in lead $V_6$ (Fig. 9.12). The left ventricle is depolarized normally via the left bundle branch, causing an S wave in lead $V_1$ and an R wave in lead $V_6$ (Fig. 9.13). Then, the right ventricle is depolarized by the left, causing another R wave (called R') in lead $V_1$ and an S wave in lead $V_6$ (Fig. 9.14).

RBBB is discussed further in Chapter 14 (p. 153).

AN AIDE-MÉMOIRE

Remembering the name 'William Marrow' should help you recall that:

• In LBBB, the QRS looks like a 'W' in lead $V_1$ and an 'M' in lead $V_6$ (William).
• In RBBB, the QRS looks like an 'M' in lead $V_1$ and a 'W' in lead $V_6$ (Marrow).

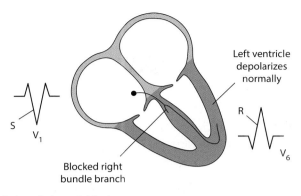

**Figure 9.13** Right bundle branch block – step two.

Key point:  • The left ventricle depolarizes normally, leading to an S wave in lead V₁ and an R wave in lead V₆.

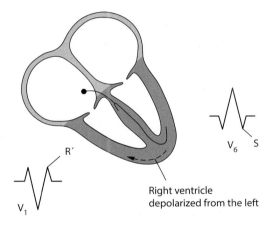

**Figure 9.14** Right bundle branch block – step three.

Key point:  • The right ventricle depolarizes late (via the left ventricle), leading to an R' wave in lead V₁ and an S wave in lead V₆.

## CONDUCTION BLOCK AT THE FASCICLES

The left bundle doesn't have to be blocked in its entirety. Instead, just one of its fascicles (anterior or posterior) may become blocked (Fig. 9.1). When this occurs, it is known as a fascicular block (or 'hemiblock').

## Left anterior fascicular block

Block of the anterior fascicle of the left bundle branch is known as left anterior fascicular block (LAFB). On the ECG, the primary consequence of LAFB is left axis deviation. LAFB is discussed in more detail in Chapter 10 (p. 114).

## Left posterior fascicular block

Block of the posterior fascicle of the left bundle branch is known as left posterior fascicular block (LPFB), and this is much less common than LAFB. On the ECG, the primary consequence of LPFB is right axis deviation. LPFB is discussed in more detail in Chapter 10 (p. 117).

### COMBINATIONS OF CONDUCTION BLOCKS

Conduction abnormalities can occur in different permutations:

- LAFB + LPFB = LBBB
- RBBB + LAFB = bifascicular block
- RBBB + LPFB = bifascicular block
- RBBB + LAFB + first-degree AV block = trifascicular block
- RBBB + LPFB + first-degree AV block = trifascicular block
- RBBB + LBBB = third-degree AV block (complete heart block)
- RBBB + LAFB + LPFB = third-degree AV block (complete heart block)

### RATE-RELATED CONDUCTION DISTURBANCES

Conduction disturbances can sometimes be rate-dependent, only occurring at fast heart rates when compromised regions of the conducting system fail to keep pace with the conduction of impulses. This is not uncommonly seen during supraventricular tachycardia (SVT), and the resultant broad complexes can lead to an incorrect diagnosis of ventricular tachycardia (VT) by the unwary. For help in distinguishing between VT and SVT, see page 86.

## ESCAPE RHYTHMS

Escape rhythms are a form of 'safety net' for the heart and appear when there is a failure of normal impulse generation or conduction. Without escape rhythms, a complete failure of impulse generation or conduction would lead to ventricular asystole and death. Instead, the heart has a number of subsidiary pacemakers that can take over if normal impulse generation or conduction fails. The subsidiary pacemakers are located in the AV junction (AV node/bundle of His) and in the ventricular myocardium.

If the AV junction fails to receive impulses, as a result of SA block or sinus arrest, or even during severe sinus bradycardia, it will take over as the cardiac pacemaker. The QRS complex(es) generated will have the same morphology as normal, but at a slower rate of around 40–60 beats/min. Figure 9.6 shows third-degree heart block (at the level of the AV node) with a junctional (narrow complex) escape rhythm which, because the QRS complexes are narrow, must be arising 'high up' in the conduction system, i.e. at or just below the AV node.

The AV junctional pacemaker will continue until it again starts to be inhibited by impulses from the SA node. If the AV junctional pacemaker fails, or its impulses are blocked, a ventricular pacemaker will take over. Its rhythm is even slower, at 15–40 beats/min, and the QRS complexes are broad because, arising within the ventricles, they cannot gain access to the Purkinje fibres and so conduction occurs slowly from myocyte to myocyte (Fig. 9.15).

### IMPORTANT

Because escape rhythms exist as a safety net, they must *not* be suppressed. Instead, you must identify why the escape rhythm has arisen (i.e. why normal impulse generation has failed or been blocked) and correct that underlying problem. This will usually require a pacemaker and should be discussed with a cardiologist.

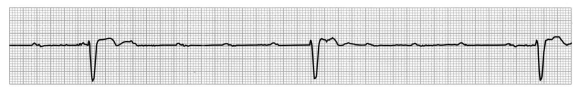

Lead II

**Figure 9.15** Third-degree AV block.

Key point:  • The P wave rate is higher than the QRS complex rate, with no relationship between them, and the QRS complexes are broad, indicating an escape rhythm arising in the ventricles.

## ACCELERATED CONDUCTION AND ACCESSORY PATHWAYS

Conduction problems aren't confined to a slowing or blockage in the transmission of impulses. Abnormal conduction can also be seen when conduction between atria and ventricles is faster than normal, and this can act as a substrate for re-entry tachycardias.

Conditions in which unusually rapid AV conduction is seen include those where there is an accessory pathway, such as Wolff–Parkinson–White (WPW) syndrome and Lown–Ganong–Levine (LGL) syndrome, and also where conduction within the AV node itself is intrinsically faster than usual (accelerated AV nodal conduction). These conditions are discussed further in Chapter 12, and the re-entry arrhythmias that can result from WPW and LGL syndrome are discussed in Chapter 7.

### SUMMARY

Problems with conduction can occur at four key points:

- SA node
  - SA block
- AV node or bundle of His
  - first-degree AV block
  - second-degree AV block
    - Mobitz type I AV block
    - Mobitz type II AV block
    - 2:1 AV block
  - third-degree AV block
- left or right bundle branches
  - LBBB
  - RBBB
- left anterior or posterior fascicles
  - LAFB
  - LPFB.

*(Continued)*

(*Continued*)

Escape rhythms occur when there is failure of normal impulse generation or conduction, and can arise from the:

- AV junction (AV node/bundle of His)
- ventricular myocardium.

Conduction problems also include accelerated conduction, as seen in:

- WPW syndrome
- LGL syndrome
- accelerated AV nodal conduction.

## FURTHER READING

Barold SS, Hayes DL. Second-degree atrioventricular block: a reappraisal. *Mayo Clinic Proceedings* 2001; **76**: 44–57.

Epstein AE, DiMarco JP, Ellenbogen KA *et al*. ACC/AHA/HRS 2008 guidelines for device based therapy of cardiac rhythm abnormalities. A Report of the American College of Cardiology/American Heart Association task force on practice guidelines (writing committee to revise the ACC/AHA/NASPE 2002 guideline update for implantation of cardiac pacemakers and antiarrhythmia devices). *J Am Coll Cardiol* 2008; **51**: e1–62.

The Task Force for Cardiac Pacing and Cardiac Resynchronization Therapy of the European Society of Cardiology. Guidelines for cardiac pacing and cardiac resynchronization therapy. *Eur Heart J* 2007; **28**: 2256–2295.

# CHAPTER 10

# The axis

Working out the QRS (or 'cardiac') axis causes more confusion than almost any other aspect of ECG assessment. This should not really be the case, as there is no mystery to the QRS axis and it is usually straightforward to assess. Indeed, deciding whether the QRS axis is normal can be summarized in one rule.

---

### A QUICK RULE FOR ASSESSING THE AXIS

If the QRS complexes are predominantly positive in leads I and II, the QRS axis is normal.

---

If you are confident about assessing the axis, you can go straight to the second half of this chapter, where we explain the causes of an abnormal axis. If not, read through the first half of the chapter, where we explain in straightforward terms what the axis represents and how it can be measured.

## UNDERSTANDING AND MEASURING THE QRS AXIS

### What does the axis mean?

As we explained earlier in this book, the flow of electrical current through the heart is fairly uniform, as it normally passes along a well-defined pathway (Fig. 10.1).

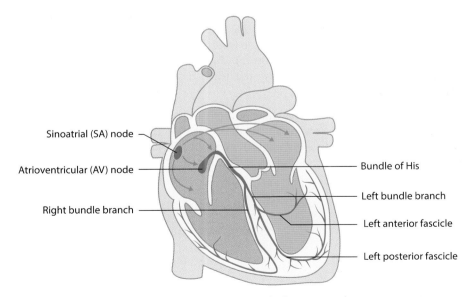

Sinoatrial (SA) node

Atrioventricular (AV) node

Right bundle branch

Bundle of His

Left bundle branch

Left anterior fascicle

Left posterior fascicle

**Figure 10.1** The flow of electrical impulses through the heart.

Key point:
• Impulses originate in the sinoatrial node, and reach the ventricles via the atrioventricular node.

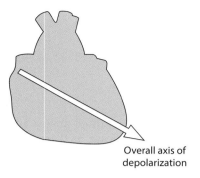

**Figure 10.2** The general direction of flow of electrical current through the heart.

Key point:
- Flow starts at the 'top right hand corner' and is towards the 'bottom left hand corner'.

Overall axis of depolarization

In simple terms, the QRS axis is an indicator of the general direction that the wave of depolarization takes as it flows through the ventricles – in other words, the overall vector of ventricular depolarization. If you think just about the general direction of electrical current as it flows through the ventricles, it starts at the base of the heart and flows towards the apex (Fig. 10.2).

## What measurement is used for the axis?

When describing the axis, a more precise terminology is required. The QRS axis is therefore conventionally referred to as the angle, measured in degrees, of the direction of electrical current flowing through the ventricles.

The reference, or zero, point is taken as a horizontal line 'looking' at the heart from the left (Fig. 10.3). For a direction of flow directed below the line, the angle is expressed as a positive number; above the line, as a negative number (Fig. 10.4). Thus, the axis can be either +1° to +180°, or –1° to –180°.

You will remember from Chapter 2 that the six limb leads look at the heart in the frontal (also called coronal) plane from six different viewpoints. The same reference system can be used to describe the angle from which each lead looks at the heart – this is represented by a **hexaxial diagram** (Fig. 10.5), which visually represents the angle from which each limb lead views the heart. The limb leads and their angles are listed in Table 10.1.

Make an effort to remember the viewpoint of each limb lead now, by learning the hexaxial diagram, before reading any further. Once you have grasped the concept of each limb lead having a different angle of view of the heart, understanding the axis will be easy.

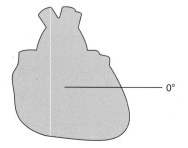

0°

**Figure 10.3** The reference (or 'zero') point for axis measurements.

Key points:
- The zero point is a horizontal line looking at the heart from the left.
- This is the same as the viewpoint of lead I.
- All axis measurements are made relative to this line.

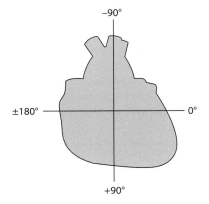

**Figure 10.4** The range of angles of the QRS axis.

Key points:  • Anticlockwise measurements are negative, clockwise measurements are positive.
 • All measurements are relative to the zero line.

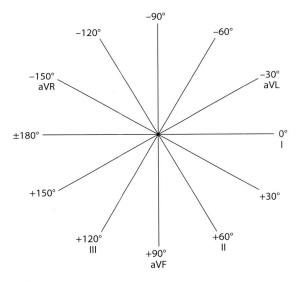

**Fig. 10.5** Viewpoints of the six limb leads.

Key point:  • Each lead 'looks' at the heart from a different angle.

**Table 10.1** Limb leads and angles of view

| Limb lead | Angle at which it views the heart |
|-----------|-----------------------------------|
| I | 0° |
| II | +60° |
| III | +120° |
| aVR | −150° |
| aVL | −30° |
| aVF | +90° |

## How do I use the limb leads to work out the axis?

The information from the limb leads is used to work out the QRS axis. Simply remember three principles, all of which we have covered already:

1. The QRS axis is the general direction of electrical flow through the ventricles.

> ## WHAT IS A 'NORMAL' AXIS?
>
> Unfortunately, there is no universal agreement on what is a normal QRS axis. For the purposes of this book, we consider a normal axis to be anything between −30° and +90°, although we should mention that some cardiologists accept anything up to +120° as normal. This is because there is no definitive dividing line between normality and abnormality. The most sensible approach is to consider that the likelihood of a patient having an underlying abnormality increases as the axis increases from +90° to +120°.

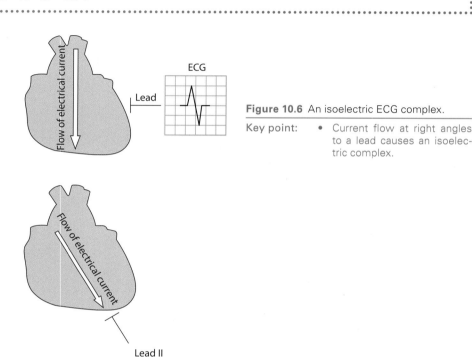

**Figure 10.6** An isoelectric ECG complex.

Key point:
- Current flow at right angles to a lead causes an isoelectric complex.

**Figure 10.7** The QRS complex is positive in lead II.

Key points:
- Flow towards a lead causes a positive deflection.
- Current flow in the ventricles is towards lead II.

2. Each of the limb leads records this electrical flow from a different viewpoint of the heart.

3. Electrical flow towards a lead causes a positive deflection, and flow away from a lead causes a negative deflection.

The last rule means that if current flows at right angles to a lead, the ECG complex generated will be isoelectric, that is, the positive and negative deflections will be equal. This is illustrated in Figure 10.6.

Using these principles, consider how lead II records ventricular depolarization. From its point of view, the flow of current in the ventricles is entirely towards it and the QRS complex is entirely positive (Fig. 10.7). Lead aVL, however, will see the same current at right angles to itself and record an isoelectric QRS complex (Fig. 10.8).

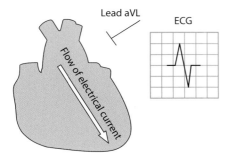

**Figure 10.8** An isoelectric QRS complex in lead aVL.

Key points:
- Flow at right angles to a lead causes an isoelectric complex.
- Current flow in this example is at right angles to lead aVL.

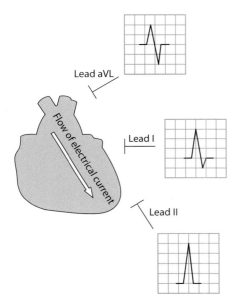

**Figure 10.9** The QRS complex is predominantly positive in lead I.

Key point:
- Lead I lies between leads II and aVL.

Any lead looking from a viewpoint between leads II and aVL will record a complex that becomes increasingly positive the closer it is to lead II (Fig. 10.9).

It should now be fairly clear that you can work out the QRS axis by examining whether the QRS complexes in the limb leads are predominantly positive or negative.

There are several ways to determine the QRS axis: some ways are quick and approximate, others are more precise but detailed.

## A quick way to work out the QRS axis

This technique enables you to decide within seconds whether the QRS axis is normal or abnormal. To decide whether the axis is normal, you need only look at two of the limb leads: I and II.

If the QRS complex in **lead I** is predominantly positive, this indicates that the axis lies anywhere between –90° and +90° (Fig. 10.10). An axis at *exactly* –90° or +90° would cause a precisely isoelectric QRS complex in lead I. Thus, a predominantly positive QRS complex in lead I rules out right axis deviation (an axis beyond +90°), but does not exclude left axis deviation (an axis beyond –30°).

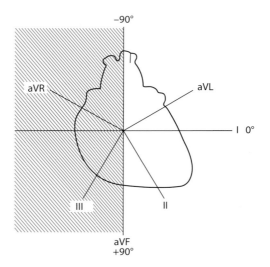

**Figure 10.10** A predominantly positive QRS in lead I puts the axis between −90° and +90°.

Key point:    • A predominantly positive QRS in lead I therefore excludes right axis deviation.

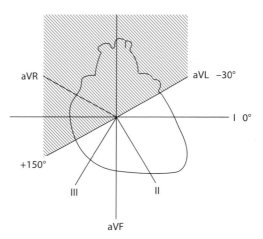

**Figure 10.11** A predominantly positive QRS in lead II puts the axis between −30° and +150°.

Key point:    • A predominantly positive QRS in lead II therefore excludes left axis deviation.

If the QRS complex in **lead II** is predominantly positive, this indicates that the axis lies anywhere between −30° and +150° (Fig. 10.11). An axis at *exactly* −30° or +150° would cause a precisely isoelectric QRS complex in lead II. Thus, a predominantly positive QRS complex in lead II rules out left axis deviation (an axis beyond −30°), but does not exclude right axis deviation (an axis beyond +90°).

Therefore, by looking at whether the QRS complex is positive or negative in both these leads, it is possible to say immediately whether the QRS axis is normal, or whether there is left or right axis deviation:

- a positive QRS complex in both leads I and II means the **axis is normal**
- a positive QRS complex in lead I and a negative QRS complex in lead II mean there is **left axis deviation**

**Table 10.2** Working out the QRS axis

| Lead I | Lead II | QRS axis |
| --- | --- | --- |
| Positive QRS | Positive QRS | Normal axis (−30° to +90°) |
| Positive QRS | Negative QRS | Left axis deviation (−30° to −90°) |
| Negative QRS | Positive QRS | Right axis deviation (+90° to ±180°) |
| Negative QRS | Negative QRS | Extreme right axis deviation (−90° to ±180°) |

- a negative QRS complex in lead I and a positive QRS complex in lead II mean there is **right axis deviation**
- a negative QRS complex in lead I and a negative QRS complex in lead II mean there is **extreme right axis deviation**.

These rules are summarized in Table 10.2.

When you assess the QRS axis, ask the following questions:

- Is there left axis deviation?
- Is there right axis deviation?
- Is there extreme right axis deviation?

The causes of these abnormalities, with guidance on their management, are discussed in the second half of this chapter.

### AN ALTERNATIVE QUICK METHOD

Another commonly used method for QRS axis assessment is to look for a limb lead in which the QRS complex is isoelectric (also known as 'equiphasic') – i.e. the R wave and S wave are of equal size. The overall vector of current flow must be at right angles to this lead. For instance, in Figure 10.12 the QRS complex in lead III is isoelectric. Lead III looks at the heart from an angle of +120°, so we can conclude that the QRS axis must lie at right angles to this lead, i.e. the QRS axis must be either +30° or +210°. To work out which of these is correct, look at the leads adjacent to the one you have just used – in this case, look at leads aVF and aVR. If the axis lies to the left of lead III (i.e. +30°), then the QRS will be positive in the lead to the left (aVF). If the axis lies to the right of lead III (i.e. +210°), then the QRS complex will be positive in the lead to the right (aVR). In Figure 10.12, the QRS is positive in aVF (and, as you would therefore expect, is negative in aVR). You can therefore deduce that the QRS axis must lie at +30°.

## A more precise way to calculate the QRS axis

For most practical purposes, it is not necessary to determine precisely the QRS axis of the heart – it is sufficient to know simply whether the axis is normal or abnormal. Calculating the axis precisely is not difficult but does take a little time, and this section explains how.

The method relies on the use of vectors and knowledge of how to calculate angles in right-angled triangles. Begin by finding two leads that look at the heart at right angles to each other, for example leads I and aVF (Fig. 10.12).

Next, look at the QRS complexes in these leads in Figure 10.13 and work out their overall sizes and polarities by subtracting the depth of the S wave from the height of the R wave. The overall QRS 'height' is +7 mm in lead I, and +4 mm in lead aVF.

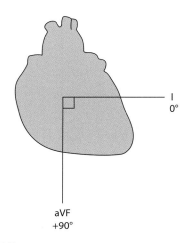

**Figure 10.12** Leads I and aVF.

Key point:    • Leads I and aVF are at right angles to each other.

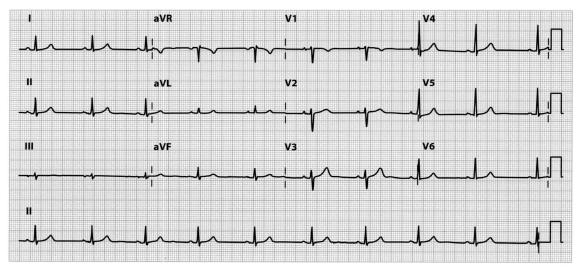

**Figure 10.13** 12-lead ECG.

Key point:    • The QRS axis is normal at +30°.

The polarity (positive or negative) of the QRS complex tells you whether the impulse is moving towards or away from the lead. The overall size tells you how much of the electricity is flowing in that direction. Using this information, you can construct a vector diagram (Fig. 10.14).

Thus, by combining the information from the two leads, you can use a pocket calculator to work out the angle at which the current is flowing (i.e. the QRS axis).

**REMEMBER**

- Sine of an angle = opposite edge/hypotenuse
- Cosine of an angle = adjacent edge/hypotenuse
- Tangent of an angle = opposite edge/adjacent edge

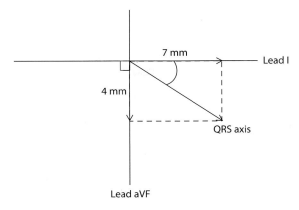

**Figure 10.14** Constructing a vector diagram.

Key points:
- Draw arrows to represent the QRS 'heights' from Figure 10.13.
- The QRS axis lies between the arrows.
- Use sine, cosine or tangent to work out the exact angle of the axis.

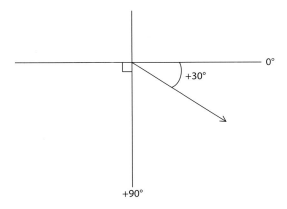

**Figure 10.15** Working out the QRS axis.

Key point:
- Do not forget to add or subtract units of 90° according to which quadrant the axis lies in.

Thus, we finally arrive at an angle in degrees (Fig. 10.15). Do not forget that the axis is measured relative to lead I, and to add or subtract units of 90° accordingly. The QRS axis in the patient in Figure 10.13 is therefore +30°, and he or she therefore has a normal QRS axis. We recommend that you practise this technique to become fully familiar with it.

### P AND T WAVE AXES

So far, we have concentrated on the axis of depolarization as measured from the QRS complexes and, although this is often referred to as the 'cardiac' axis, it is just assessing depolarization in the ventricles. However, it is also possible to work out an axis for atrial depolarization (by applying the vector analysis we have described to P waves) and for ventricular repolarization (using T waves). These measurements are seldom necessary, except where a more detailed analysis of the ECG is required.

## IS THERE LEFT AXIS DEVIATION?

Left axis deviation is present when the QRS axis lies beyond –30°. This sometimes occurs in normal individuals, but more often indicates one of the following:

- left anterior fascicular block
- Wolff–Parkinson–White (WPW) syndrome
- inferior myocardial infarction
- ventricular tachycardia.

These are discussed below.

Left ventricular hypertrophy can cause left axis deviation but *not* as a result of increased muscle mass (unlike right ventricular hypertrophy). Instead, it results from left anterior fascicular block caused by fibrosis. Contrary to some textbooks, neither obesity nor pregnancy causes left axis deviation (although obesity can cause a *leftward shift* with the axis staying within normal limits).

### Left anterior fascicular block

In Chapter 1, we describe how electrical impulses are conducted within the inter-ventricular septum in the left and right bundle branches, and that the left bundle branch divides into anterior and posterior fascicles (Fig. 10.1). Either (or both) of these fascicles can become blocked. Block of the left anterior fascicle is called left anterior fascicular block (or 'left anterior hemiblock'), and is the commonest cause of left axis deviation (Fig. 10.16).

Left anterior fascicular block can occur as a result of fibrosis of the conducting system (of any cause) or from myocardial infarction. On its own, it is not thought to carry any prognostic significance. However, left anterior fascicular block in combination with right bundle branch block (p. 153) means that two of the three main conducting pathways to the ventricles are blocked. This is termed **bifascicular block** (Fig. 10.17).

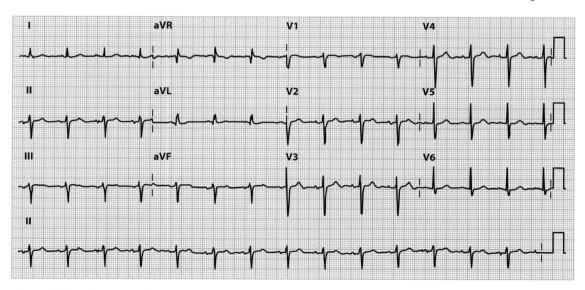

**Figure 10.16** Left axis deviation.

Key point:    • The QRS is positive in lead I and negative in lead II. The QRS axis is –56°.

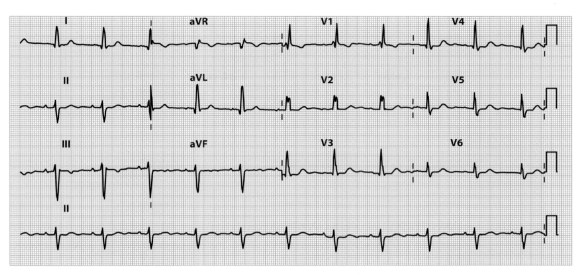

**Figure 10.17** Bifascicular block.

Key points:
- There is left axis deviation (QRS axis is −54°) together with right bundle branch block.
- The PR interval is normal.

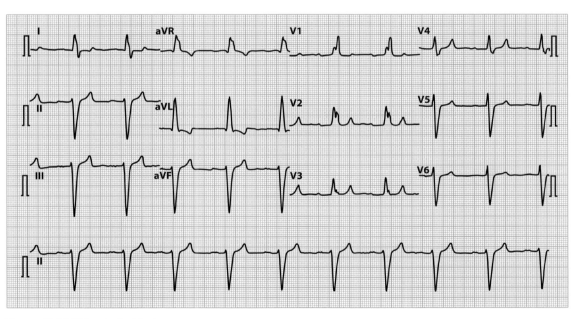

**Figure 10.18** Trifascicular block.

Key point:
- There is left axis deviation (QRS axis is −81°) together with right bundle branch block and first-degree AV block (PR interval is 266 msec).

Block of the conducting pathways can occur in any combination. A block of both fascicles is the equivalent of left bundle branch block. Block of the right bundle branch and either fascicle is bifascicular block. If bifascicular block is combined with first-degree AV block (long PR interval), this is called **trifascicular block** (Fig. 10.18).

Block of the right bundle branch and both fascicles leaves no route for impulses to reach the ventricles, and this is the equivalent of third-degree ('complete') AV block (p. 96).

Bifascicular or trifascicular block in a patient with syncopal episodes is often sufficient indication for a permanent pacemaker, even if higher degrees of block have not been documented. You should therefore refer these patients to a cardiologist. *Asymptomatic* bifascicular block, or even trifascicular block, is not necessarily an indication for pacing – discuss with a cardiologist.

**SEEK HELP**

Bifascicular or trifascicular block with syncope usually requires pacing. Referral to a cardiologist is recommended.

### Wolff–Parkinson–White syndrome

Patients with Wolff–Parkinson–White (WPW) syndrome have an accessory pathway that bypasses the atrioventricular node and bundle of His to connect the atria directly to the ventricles. If this pathway lies between the atria and ventricles on the right side of the heart, patients may have left axis deviation in addition to the other ECG appearances of WPW syndrome (discussed on p. 69).

### Inferior myocardial infarction

Left axis deviation may be a feature of myocardial infarction affecting the inferior aspect of the heart (the QRS axis is directed away from infarcted areas). The diagnosis will usually be apparent from the presentation and other ECG findings. For more information on the diagnosis and treatment of acute myocardial infarction, see Chapter 9.

### Ventricular tachycardia (with a focus in the left ventricular apex)

When ventricular tachycardia arises from a focus in the left ventricular apex, the wave of depolarization spreads out through the rest of the myocardium from that point, resulting in left axis deviation. The diagnosis and treatment of ventricular tachycardia are discussed on page 83.

## IS THERE RIGHT AXIS DEVIATION?

Right axis deviation is present when the QRS axis lies beyond +90° (Fig. 10.19). This sometimes occurs in normal individuals, but more often indicates one of the following:

- right ventricular hypertrophy
- WPW syndrome
- anterolateral myocardial infarction
- dextrocardia
- left posterior fascicular block.

### Right ventricular hypertrophy

Right ventricular hypertrophy is the commonest cause of right axis deviation. Other ECG evidence of right ventricular hypertrophy includes:

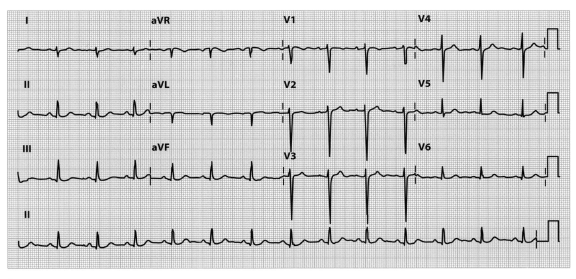

**Figure 10.19** Right axis deviation.

Key points:
- The QRS is negative in lead I and positive in lead II.
- The QRS axis is +98°.

- dominant R wave in lead V$_1$
- deep S waves in leads V$_5$ and V$_6$
- right bundle branch block.

For more information on the causes of right ventricular hypertrophy, turn to page 147.

## Wolff–Parkinson–White syndrome

As with right-sided accessory pathways and left axis deviation, patients with WPW syndrome who have a left-sided accessory pathway may have right axis deviation in addition to the other ECG appearances of WPW syndrome. WPW syndrome is discussed in more detail on page 67.

## Anterolateral myocardial infarction

The QRS axis is directed away from infarcted areas. Thus, right axis deviation may be a feature of anterolateral myocardial infarction. The diagnosis will usually be apparent from the presentation and other ECG findings. For more information on the diagnosis and treatment of acute myocardial infarction, see Chapter 15.

## Dextrocardia

Right axis deviation is a feature of dextrocardia (in which the heart lies on the right side of the chest instead of the left), but the most obvious abnormality is that all the chest leads have 'right ventricular' QRS complexes (see Fig. 14.6, p. 150). Dextrocardia is discussed in more detail on page 149.

## Left posterior fascicular block

Unlike left anterior fascicular block, left posterior fascicular block is extremely rare. It is identified in approximately only 1 in 10,000 ECGs. It is therefore extremely important that if you identify right axis deviation on an ECG, you rule out other causes (in particular, right ventricular hypertrophy) before diagnosing left posterior fascicular block. The causes and management of left posterior fascicular block are the same as for left anterior fascicular block (p. 114).

## IS THERE EXTREME RIGHT AXIS DEVIATION?

Extreme right axis deviation is present when the QRS axis lies between −90° and ±180°. This is uncommonly due to a clinical cause, and most frequently occurs when there has been misplacement of the ECG electrodes – thus if you see extreme right axis deviation, always double check whether the limb electrodes were placed correctly.

If extreme right axis deviation is present, then possible causes include:

- ventricular tachycardia with extreme axis shift (p. 83)
- ventricular pacing (p. 209).

## SUMMARY

Quick rule: If the QRS complexes are predominantly positive in leads I and II, the QRS axis is normal. To assess the QRS axis, ask the following questions:

*1. Is there left axis deviation?*

If 'yes', consider:

- left anterior fascicular block
- WPW syndrome
- inferior myocardial infarction
- ventricular tachycardia (with left ventricular apical focus).

*2. Is there right axis deviation?*

If 'yes', consider:

- right ventricular hypertrophy
- WPW syndrome
- anterolateral myocardial infarction
- dextrocardia
- left posterior fascicular block.

*3. Is there extreme right axis deviation?*

If 'yes', consider:

- limb electrode misplacement
- ventricular tachycardia
- ventricular pacing.

## FURTHER READING

Meek S, Morri F. ABC of clinical electrocardiography: Introduction. I – Leads, rate, rhythm, and cardiac axis. *Br Med J* 2002; **324**: 415–418.

After determining the heart rate, rhythm and axis, examine each wave of the ECG in turn, beginning with the P wave. You may already have noticed abnormal P waves while assessing the cardiac rhythm, but in this chapter we tell you how to examine the P wave in more detail and what abnormalities to look out for.

As you examine the P wave in each lead, the questions to ask are:

- Are any P waves absent?
- Are any P waves inverted?
- Are any P waves too tall?
- Are any P waves too wide?

> **THE ORIGIN OF THE P WAVE**
>
> You will recall from Chapter 2 that the P wave represents atrial depolarization. It does not, as some people mistakenly believe, represent sinoatrial (SA) node depolarization; it is possible to have P waves without SA node depolarization (e.g. atrial ectopics) or SA node depolarization without P waves (SA block).

## ARE ANY P WAVES ABSENT?

The SA node is normally a regular and dependable natural pacemaker. Atrial depolarization (and thus P wave formation) is therefore normally so regular that it is easy to predict when the next P wave is going to appear (Fig. 11.1).

The only normal circumstance in which the P wave rate is variable is sinus arrhythmia, which is usually only seen in patients below the age of 40 years. Sinus arrhythmia is discussed on page 54.

In this section, we tell you what diagnoses to consider if you find that P waves are absent. By this, we mean that they can be either:

- completely absent (no P waves on the whole ECG), or
- intermittently absent (some P waves do not appear where expected).

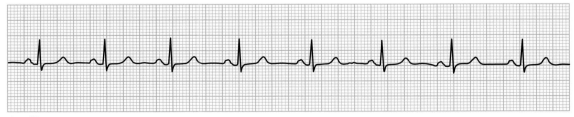

Lead II

**Figure 11.1** Sinus rhythm.

Key point: • The P waves are regular and it's therefore easy to predict when the next P wave will appear.

## P waves are completely absent

There are two reasons why P waves may be absent from the ECG. The first is that there is no coordinated atrial depolarization so that P waves are not being formed. The second is that P waves *are* present, but are just not obvious.

A lack of coordinated atrial depolarization occurs in atrial fibrillation, and this is the commonest reason for P waves to be truly absent from the ECG (Fig. 11.2). Instead of P waves, the chaotic atrial activity produces low-amplitude oscillations (fibrillation or 'f' waves) on the ECG. Atrial fibrillation can be recognized by the absence of P waves and the erratic occurrence of QRS complexes. Atrial fibrillation is discussed on page 59.

P waves will also be completely absent if there is a prolonged period of sinus arrest or sinoatrial block. In these conditions, atrial activation does not occur because the SA node either fails to depolarize (sinus arrest) or fails to transmit the depolarization to the atria (SA block). Either condition *can* cause ventricular asystole, but more commonly an escape rhythm takes over (Fig. 11.3). See page 94 for more information on sinus arrest and SA block.

Absent P waves are also one of the possible ECG manifestations of hyperkalaemia (p. 180). If this is a possibility, look for associated ECG abnormalities and check the patient's plasma potassium level urgently.

It is very common for P waves to be present but not immediately obvious. Search the ECG carefully for evidence of P waves before concluding that they are absent, as P waves will often be hidden by any rapid tachycardia (Fig. 11.4). In normal sinus rhythm the P waves are usually best seen in leads II and $V_1$, and so examine these leads particularly closely. P waves may also occasionally be hidden within the QRS complexes or T waves in third degree AV block (Fig. 11.5) and in AV dissociation (Fig. 12.10).

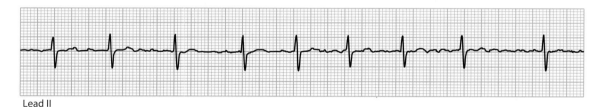

Lead II

**Figure 11.2** Atrial fibrillation.

Key point:   • The P waves are absent (no obvious coordinated atrial activity) and there is an erratic ('irregularly irregular') QRS rhythm.

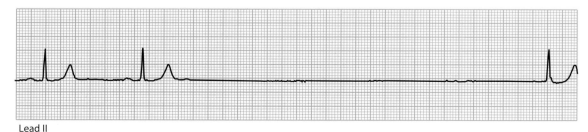

Lead II

**Figure 11.3** Sinus pause followed by a junctional escape beat.

Key points:   • After two sinus beats there is a prolonged pause, lasting almost 5.5 s, with no P wave activity.
   • This is followed by a junctional escape beat.

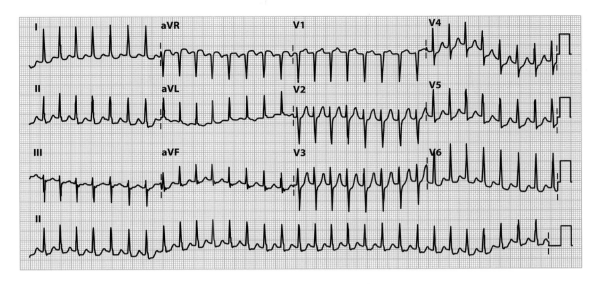

**Figure 11.4** AV nodal re-entry tachycardia.

Key point:
- P waves can just be discerned as a small deflection immediately after the end of the QRS complexes in some leads.

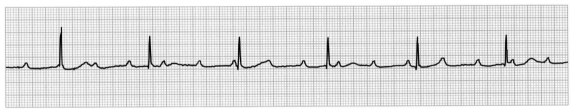

Lead II

**Figure 11.5** Third-degree AV block.

Key point:
- The P waves occasionally merge with the QRS complexes or T waves, and are therefore 'hidden' by them.

Even in sinus tachycardia, at high heart rates the P waves may start to overlap with the T waves of the previous beats, making them hard to identify.

At very high atrial rates, such as in atrial flutter, P waves may not be apparent because they become distorted. In atrial flutter, the atria usually depolarize around 300 times/min. The P waves generated by this rapid activity are called flutter waves, and have a 'sawtooth' appearance. Atrial flutter is discussed on page 64.

In ventricular tachycardia, retrograde (backward) conduction up through the AV node may cause each QRS complex to be *followed* by a P wave which may not be immediately obvious and which also, incidentally, will be inverted. Even more importantly, *independent* atrial activity can occur during ventricular tachycardia, and the P waves can be buried anywhere within the QRS complexes (p. 87). Evidence of independent atrial activity is a very useful clue in the differentiation of ventricular and supraventricular tachycardias.

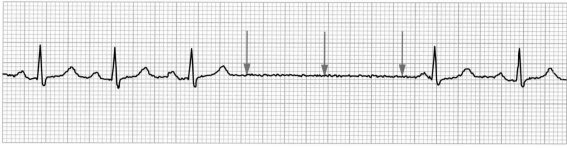

Lead II

**Figure 11.6** Sinus arrest.

### P waves are intermittently absent

The SA node is usually an extremely reliable natural pacemaker. The occasional absence of a P wave on an ECG indicates that the SA node has either failed to generate an impulse (sinus arrest, Fig. 11.6) or failed to conduct the impulse to the surrounding atrial tissue (SA block). For examples of both these conditions, together with guidance on how to distinguish them, see page 94.

## ARE ANY P WAVES INVERTED?

The P wave is usually upright in all leads except aVR, which 'looks' at the atria from roughly the patient's right shoulder and so detects the wave of atrial depolarization moving away from it (Fig. 2.9). The P wave may sometimes be inverted in lead $V_1$ also, although it is more usually biphasic in that lead (Fig. 11.7).

Whenever you see an inverted P wave, ask yourself:

● Were the electrodes correctly positioned?

Abnormal P wave inversion can indicate either of the following:

● dextrocardia

● abnormal atrial depolarization.

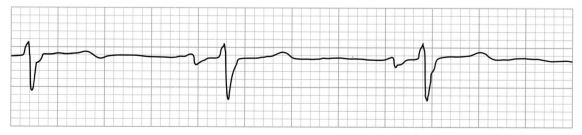

Lead V1

**Figure 11.7** Biphasic P wave.

Key point:   •  The P wave is normally biphasic in lead $V_1$.

Dextrocardia is discussed on page 149. Abnormal atrial depolarization is explained below.

## Abnormal atrial depolarization

The wave of depolarization normally spreads through the atria from the SA node to the AV node. If atrial depolarization is initiated from within, near or through the AV node, the wave will travel in the opposite (retrograde) direction through the atria. From the 'viewpoints' of most of the ECG leads, this wave will be moving *away from* rather than towards them, and *inverted* P waves will be produced (see Fig. 11.4).

Many abnormal sources of atrial activation can thus cause retrograde depolarization and inverted P waves, including:

- atrial ectopics
- AV junctional rhythms
- ventricular tachycardia (retrogradely conducted)
- ventricular ectopics (retrogradely conducted).

## ARE ANY P WAVES TOO TALL?

Normal P waves are usually less than 0.25 mV (2.5 small squares) in amplitude. Tall, peaked P waves indicate right atrial enlargement. The abnormality is sometimes referred to as 'P pulmonale', because right atrial enlargement is often secondary to pulmonary disorders. An example is shown in Figure 11.8. If the P waves appear unusually tall, assess your patient for any of the causes of right atrial enlargement (Table 11.1).

Abnormally tall P waves should draw attention to the possibility of an underlying disorder that may require further investigation. In addition to a thorough patient history and examination, a chest radiograph (to assess cardiac dimensions and lung fields) and an echocardiogram (to assess valvular disorders and estimate pulmonary artery pressure) may be helpful.

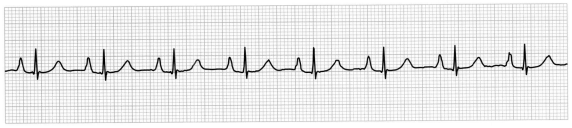

Lead II

**Figure 11.8** P pulmonale.

Key point:    • Tall P waves (3.5 mm in lead II).

**Table 11.1** Causes of right atrial enlargement

- Primary pulmonary hypertension
- Secondary pulmonary hypertension
  - chronic bronchitis
  - emphysema
  - massive pulmonary embolism
- Pulmonary stenosis
- Tricuspid stenosis

## ARE ANY P WAVES TOO WIDE?

Normal P waves are usually less than 0.12 s (3 small squares) in duration. Minor notching of the P wave ('bifid' P wave) is not uncommon, indicating a mild degree of asynchrony between right and left atrial depolarization, but any broadening of the P wave with a notch greater than 0.1 mV (1 small square) in depth should arouse suspicion of left atrial enlargement. This is usually a result of mitral valve disease, and consequently these broad, bifid P waves are known as 'P mitrale' (Fig. 11.9).

The P wave becomes broad because the enlarged left atrium takes longer than normal to depolarize. As with P pulmonale, P mitrale does not require treatment in its own right, but should alert you to a possible underlying problem. This is often mitral valve disease, but left atrial enlargement can also accompany left ventricular hypertrophy (e.g. secondary to hypertension, aortic valve disease and hypertrophic cardiomyopathy). A chest X-ray and an echocardiogram may be helpful following a patient history and examination.

### P WAVE DISPERSION

The duration of the P wave has attracted research interest. Prolongation of P wave duration and also increased P wave dispersion (the difference between P wave durations in different leads in the 12-lead ECG) have been identified as predictors of risk for the development of atrial fibrillation.

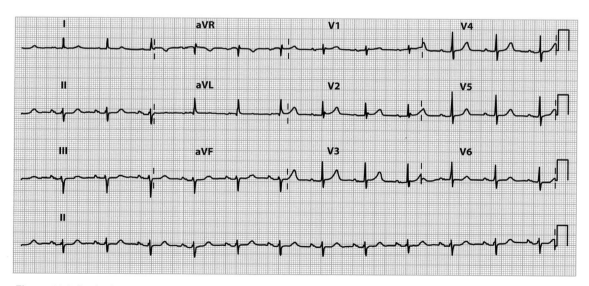

**Figure 11.9** P mitrale.

Key point:    • The P waves are broad and bifid.

## SUMMARY

To assess the P wave, ask the following questions:

*1. Are any P waves absent?*

If 'yes', consider:

- P waves are completely absent
  - atrial fibrillation
  - sinus arrest or SA block (prolonged)
  - hyperkalaemia
- P waves are present but not obvious
- P waves are intermittently absent
  - sinus arrest or SA block (intermittent).

*2. Are any P waves inverted?*

If 'yes', consider:

- electrode misplacement
- dextrocardia
- retrograde atrial depolarization.

*3. Are any P waves too tall?*

If 'yes', consider:

- right atrial enlargement.

*4. Are any P waves too wide?*

If 'yes', consider:

- left atrial enlargement.

## FURTHER READING

Dilaveris PE, Gialafos JE. P-wave dispersion: a novel predictor of paroxysmal atrial fibrillation. *Annals of Noninvasive Electrocardiology* 2001; **6**: 159–165.

Hurst JW. Naming of the waves in the ECG, with a brief account of their genesis. *Circulation* 1998; **98**: 1937–1942.

# CHAPTER 12

# The PR interval

Once the sinus node has generated an electrical stimulus, this must be transmitted through the atria, atrioventricular (AV) node and bundle of His to reach the ventricles and bring about cardiac contraction. The time delay while this occurs is mainly taken up by the passage of the electrical impulse through the AV node, which acts as a regulator of conduction. This corresponds to the PR interval on the ECG (Fig. 12.1).

The PR interval has precise time limits. In health, this interval is:

- no less than 0.12 s (3 small squares) long
- no more than 0.2 s (5 small squares) long
- consistent in length.

Make sure you check the duration of as many consecutive PR intervals as you can and ask the following questions:

- Is the PR interval less than 0.12 s long?
- Is the PR interval more than 0.2 s long?
- Does the PR interval vary or can it not be measured?
- Is the PR segment elevated or depressed?

This chapter will help you to answer these questions and to reach a diagnosis if you find any abnormalities.

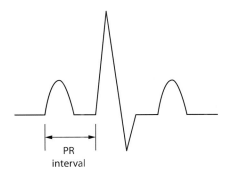

**Figure 12.1** The PR interval.

Key point:　• This is measured from the start of the P wave to the start of the R wave.

## IS THE PR INTERVAL LESS THAN 0.12 S LONG?

A PR interval of less than 0.12 s (3 small squares) indicates that the usual delay to conduction between the atria and the ventricles, imposed by the AV junction, has not occurred. This happens if depolarization *originates* in the AV junction, so that it travels up to the atria and down to the ventricles simultaneously, or if it originates as normal in the sinus node but bypasses the AV junction via an *additional faster-conducting pathway*.

A short PR interval should therefore prompt you to think of:

- AV nodal rhythm
- Wolff–Parkinson–White (WPW) syndrome
- Lown–Ganong–Levine (LGL) syndrome
- accelerated AV nodal conduction.

Details of how to recognize and manage each of these are given below.

## AV nodal rhythm

If depolarization is initiated from within the AV node, the wave of atrial depolarization will travel backwards through the atria at the same time as setting off forwards through the AV node towards the ventricles. Thus, the time delay between atrial depolarization (the P wave) and ventricular depolarization (the QRS complex) will be reduced (Fig. 12.2).

Any source of depolarization within the AV node can therefore cause a short PR interval, including:

- AV nodal escape rhythms
- AV ectopics
- AV re-entry tachycardia.

A discussion of how to identify and manage all of these rhythms can be found in Chapter 7. Atrial ectopics arising near to the AV node will also have a shorter PR interval than normal sinus beats, but it will rarely be less than 0.12 s long.

## Wolff–Parkinson–White syndrome

In most people, conduction of electricity through the heart follows just one distinct path from atria to ventricles, namely via the AV node, bundle of His and Purkinje fibres. Some people have an additional connection between the atria and the ventricles – an accessory pathway – that conducts more quickly than the AV

12  The PR interval

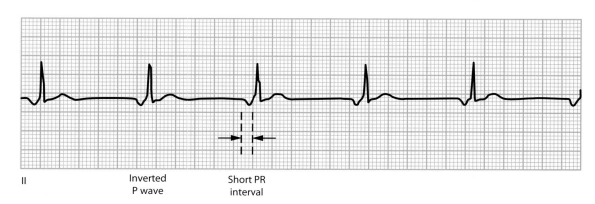

II                Inverted          Short PR
                  P wave            interval

**Figure 12.2** Depolarization from a focus in the AV node.

Key point:    • The P waves are inverted in lead II and the PR interval is abnormally short, which suggests an origin
              low in the atria near to the AV node.

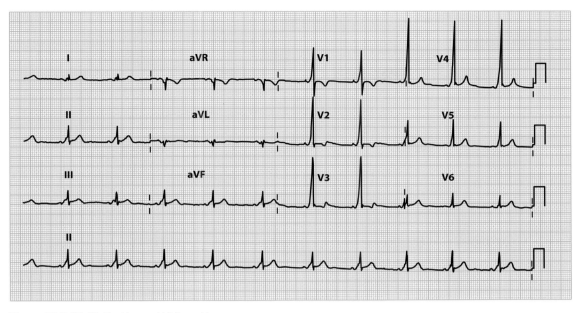

**Figure 12.3** Wolff–Parkinson–White pattern.

Key point:    • The PR interval is short and there is ventricular pre-excitation (delta wave).

node, so the wave of depolarization reaches the ventricles more quickly than usual and thus the PR interval is short.

The region of ventricle activated via the accessory pathway slowly depolarizes, giving rise to a **delta wave** – the first part of the QRS complex (Fig. 7.13). Shortly afterwards, the rest of the ventricular muscle is depolarized rapidly with the arrival of the normally conducted wave of depolarization via the AV node.

When a short PR interval and delta wave are seen on an ECG, this is called a Wolff–Parkinson–White (WPW) *pattern* (Fig. 12.3). In most cases, this is just an incidental finding and the individual has no problems with their heart rhythm. However, in some cases the presence of an accessory pathway provides a substrate for episodes of AV re-entry tachycardia (AVRT), in which case the patient is said to have WPW *syndrome*. WPW syndrome and AVRT are discussed in more detail in Chapter 7 (p. 67).

## Lown–Ganong–Levine syndrome

There has been much argument over recent years about the status of LGL syndrome and whether it truly represents a distinct pathophysiological entity.

The 'classical' view of LGL syndrome is that, like in WPW syndrome, patients have an accessory pathway (sometimes called the bundle of James) which bypasses the AV node. However, unlike the bundle of Kent in WPW syndrome, the accessory pathway in LGL syndrome does not activate the ventricular muscle directly. Instead, it simply connects the atria to the bundle of His. As a result, the AV node is bypassed (so the PR interval is short) but there is no ventricular pre-excitation (and therefore there is no delta wave).

However, short PR intervals (in the absence of a delta wave) are a relatively common finding and the contemporary view is that a short PR interval alone is not sufficient

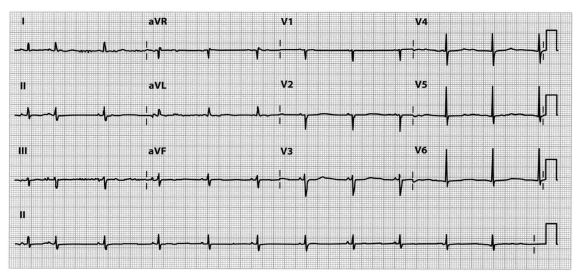

**Figure 12.4** Accelerated AV nodal conduction.

Key points:
- The PR interval is short, but there is no ventricular pre-excitation.
- This was an incidental finding in an asymptomatic individual with no history of paroxysmal tachycardias.

reason to diagnose LGL syndrome. Instead, LGL syndrome is diagnosed when patients with a short PR interval (and no delta wave) present with re-entry tachycardias. Those who do not experience re-entry tachycardias are instead considered to have a normal variant of AV conduction known as accelerated AV nodal conduction.

### DOES LGL SYNDROME ACTUALLY EXIST?

Many electrophysiologists have questioned the pathophysiological basis of LGL syndrome altogether, as a variety of fibre abnormalities have been identified quite distinct from the original description of James fibres, and the functional significance of many of these anomalies remains unclear. Indeed, most patients with a short PR interval and paroxysmal tachycardias are found to have a 'conventional' substrate for their tachycardia (such at atrioventricular nodal re-entry tachycardia) on electrophysiological testing, and it may be the case that the short PR interval simply represented an incidental variant of AV node conduction in such cases.

## Accelerated AV nodal conduction

The presence of a short PR interval in isolation, with no history of re-entry tachycardia, is regarded as a normal variant of AV node conduction (and should not be labelled as LGL syndrome). An example ECG, recorded in an asymptomatic individual, is shown in Fig. 12.4.

### IS THE PR INTERVAL MORE THAN 0.2 S LONG?

Prolongation of the PR interval is a common finding and indicates that conduction through the AV node has been delayed. When this delay is constant for each cardiac cycle, and each P wave is followed by a QRS complex, it is referred to as **first-degree AV block** (p. 94).

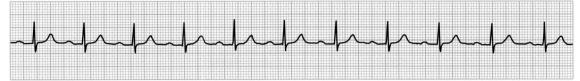

Lead II

**Figure 12.5** First-degree AV block.

Key point:    • The PR interval is prolonged, measuring 0.22 s.

First-degree AV block is a common feature of vagally induced bradycardia, as an increase in vagal tone decreases AV nodal conduction. It may also be a feature of:

- ischaemic heart disease
- hyperkalaemia or hypokalaemia
- acute rheumatic myocarditis
- Lyme disease
- drugs
- beta blockers
- rate-modifying calcium channel blockers
- digoxin.

Figure 12.5 shows a rhythm strip from a patient with first-degree AV block. Look for a cause by taking a thorough patient history and, in particular, asking about any drug treatment the patient is currently receiving.

First-degree AV block in itself is asymptomatic and, in general, does not progress to other sorts of heart block (these are described later). No specific treatment is necessary for first-degree AV block *in its own right*, but it should alert you to one of the above diagnoses (which may require treatment). First-degree AV block is *not* an indication for a pacemaker.

## DOES THE PR INTERVAL VARY OR CAN IT NOT BE MEASURED?

Normally, the PR interval is constant. In some conditions, however, the interval between P waves and QRS complexes changes, giving rise to a variable PR interval. Sometimes a P wave is not followed by a QRS complex at all and so the PR interval cannot be measured.

If either, or both, of these occur, they indicate one of several possible AV conduction problems. These are distinguished by the relationship between P waves and QRS complexes.

- If the PR interval gradually lengthens with each beat, until one P wave fails to produce a QRS complex, the patient has **Mobitz type I AV block**.
- If the PR interval is fixed and normal, but occasionally a P wave fails to produce a QRS complex, the patient has **Mobitz type II AV block**.
- If alternate P waves are not followed by QRS complexes, the patient has **2:1 AV block**.
- If there is no relationship between P waves and QRS complexes, the patient has **third-degree (complete) AV block**.

All these types of AV block are discussed below, with example ECGs.

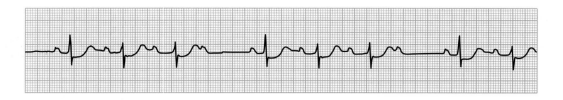

Lead II

**Figure 12.6** Mobitz type I AV block.

Key point:  • There is progressive lengthening of the PR interval, a P wave then fails to be conducted, then the PR interval 'resets' and cycle repeats.

## Mobitz type I AV block

Mobitz type I AV block is one of the types of second-degree heart block and is also known as the Wenckebach phenomenon (p. 95). Its characteristic features are:

● the PR interval shows progressive lengthening until one P wave fails to be conducted and fails to produce a QRS complex

● the PR interval resets to normal and the cycle repeats.

These features are demonstrated in the rhythm strip in Figure 12.6. When Mobitz type I AV block occurs at the level of the AV node it is generally regarded as 'benign', and a permanent pacemaker is not required unless the frequency of 'dropped' ventricular beats causes a symptomatic bradycardia. When the block is infranodal (as identified by electrophysiological testing) there is a stronger indication for pacing, even if patients are asymptomatic.

In Mobitz type I AV block in the setting of acute myocardial infarction, pacing may be required depending on the type of infarction. In **anterior** myocardial infarction, a prophylactic temporary pacemaker is recommended in case third-degree (complete) heart block develops. In **inferior** myocardial infarction, a pacemaker is only needed if symptoms or haemodynamic compromise result. Patients found to have Mobitz type I AV block prior to surgery will usually require temporary pacing perioperatively – discuss this with the anaesthetist and a cardiologist.

 **SEEK HELP**

Mobitz type I AV block may require pacing prior to surgery. Seek the advice of a cardiologist without delay.

## Mobitz type II AV block

Mobitz type II AV block is another type of second-degree heart block and its characteristic features are:

● most P waves are followed by a QRS complex

● the PR interval is normal and constant

● occasionally, a P wave is not followed by a QRS complex.

These features are demonstrated in the 12-lead ECG in Figure 12.7.

Mobitz type II AV block is thought to result from abnormal conduction below the AV node (infranodal) and is considered more serious than Mobitz type I as

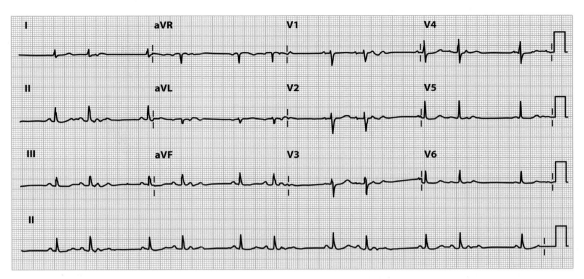

**Figure 12.7**  Mobitz type II AV block.

Key point:   • The PR interval is normal and constant, but there is an occasional failure of AV conduction and a P wave is not followed by a QRS complex.

it can progress without warning to third-degree (complete) heart block. Referral to a cardiologist is therefore recommended, as a pacemaker may be required.

The indications for pacing Mobitz type II AV block in the setting of an acute myocardial infarction, or perioperatively, are the same as for Mobitz type I AV block.

**SEEK HELP**

Mobitz type II AV block may require pacing. Seek the advice of a cardiologist without delay.

## 2:1 AV block

2:1 AV block is a special form of second-degree heart block in which alternate P waves are not followed by QRS complexes (Fig. 12.8).

2:1 AV block cannot be categorized as Mobitz type I or type II because it is impossible to say whether the PR interval for the non-conducted P waves would have been the same as, or longer than, the conducted P waves.

**SEEK HELP**

2:1 AV block usually requires pacing. Seek the advice of a cardiologist without delay.

## Third-degree AV block

In third-degree AV block ('complete heart block'), there is complete interruption of conduction between atria and ventricles, so that the two are working independently. QRS complexes usually arise as the result of a ventricular escape rhythm (p. 102). An example is shown in Figure 12.9.

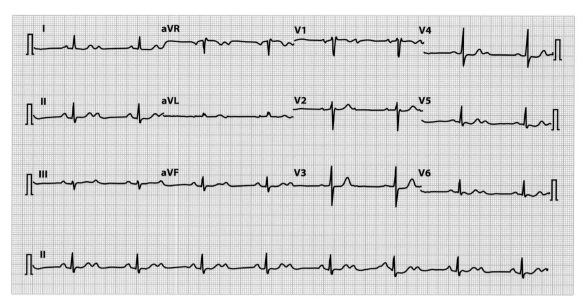

**Figure 12.8** 2:1 AV block.

Key point:    • Every alternate P wave fails to be conducted.

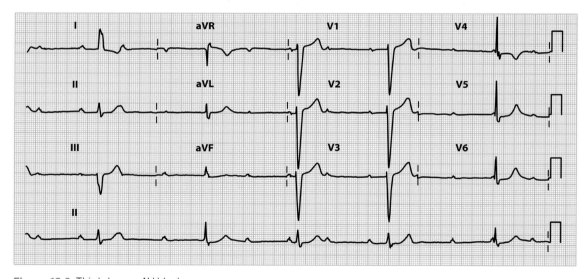

**Figure 12.9** Third-degree AV block.

Key points:    • The P wave (atrial) rate is approximately 75/min, with a QRS complex (ventricular) rate of approximately 30/min.
                • There is no relationship between P waves and QRS complexes.

The characteristic features of complete heart block are:

• P wave rate is faster than ventricular QRS complexes
• P waves bear no relationship to the ventricular QRS complexes
• if block occurs in the AV node, QRS complexes are usually narrow due to a subsidiary pacemaker arising in the bundle of His

- if block occurs below the AV node, QRS complexes are usually broad due to a subsidiary pacemaker arising in the left or right bundle branches.

It is important to remember that any atrial rhythm can coexist with third-degree AV block, and so the P waves may be abnormal or even absent. A combination of bradycardia (ventricular rate usually 15–40/min) and broad QRS complexes should alert you to suspect third-degree AV block.

In most cases, acquired third-degree AV block requires a permanent pacemaker. An exception to this is if there is a reversible cause (such as drug toxicity, e.g. beta-blockers, or infection, such as Lyme disease), in which case the patient may only require supportive treatment (which may include temporary pacing) until the cause has been treated and the AV block has resolved.

In acute **inferior** wall myocardial infarction, third-degree AV block requires temporary pacing if the patient has symptoms or is haemodynamically compromised. However, pacing may not be required if the patient is asymptomatic and has a ventricular rate >35/min. In acute **anterior** wall myocardial infarction, the development of third-degree AV block usually indicates an extensive infarct (and thus a poor prognosis) and temporary pacing is indicated regardless of the patient's symptoms or haemodynamic state. Temporary pacing is also usually necessary perioperatively in patients about to undergo surgery who are found to have third-degree AV block.

**SEEK HELP**

> Third-degree AV block usually requires pacing. Seek the advice of a cardiologist without delay.

### ATRIOVENTRICULAR DISSOCIATION

Atrioventricular dissociation is a term that is commonly used interchangeably with third-degree AV block; however, it does *not* mean the same thing. Atrioventricular dissociation occurs when the ventricular (QRS) rate is *higher* than the atrial (P wave) rate. The opposite is found in third-degree AV block. Atrioventricular dissociation usually occurs in the context of an escape rhythm (from the AV junction or ventricles) during sinus bradycardia, or an acceleration in a subsidiary focus in the AV junction or ventricles which then overtakes the sinoatrial node, which continues firing independently (Fig. 12.10).

## IS THE PR SEGMENT ELEVATED OR DEPRESSED?

The PR segment, between the end of the P wave and the start of the QRS complex, is usually flat and isoelectric. However, PR segment depression can occur in pericarditis, and is thought to be caused by atrial involvement in the inflammatory process. PR segment depression is a specific ECG feature of pericarditis and may be seen in any leads except aVR and $V_1$ (where there may be PR segment elevation). Pericarditis may also cause widespread ST segment elevation (p. 168).

PR segment depression (or, rarely, PR segment elevation) can also be seen if there is atrial involvement with an acute coronary syndrome. In the setting of acute inferior myocardial infarction, the presence of ≥1.2 mm PR segment depression is associated with worse outcomes.

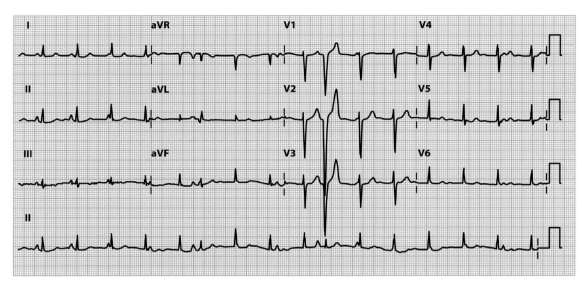

**Figure 12.10** Atrioventricular dissociation.

Key points:
- The ventricular rate (94/min) is higher than the atrial rate (approximately 80/min), causing the QRS complexes to 'march through' the P waves.
- There are also occasional incidental ventricular ectopic beats.

## SUMMARY

To assess the PR interval, ask the following questions:

*1. Is the PR interval less than 0.12 s long?*

If 'yes', consider:

- AV junctional rhythms
- WPW syndrome
- LGL syndrome
- accelerated AV nodal conduction.

*2. Is the PR interval more than 0.2 s long?*

If 'yes', consider:

- first-degree AV block
- ischaemic heart disease
- hyperkalaemia or hypokalaemia
- acute rheumatic myocarditis
- Lyme disease
- drugs (beta blockers, rate-modifying calcium channel blockers, digoxin).

*3. Does the PR interval vary or can it not be measured?*

If 'yes', consider:

- second-degree AV block
  - Mobitz type I (Wenckebach phenomenon)

*(Continued)*

(*Continued*)
- - Mobitz type II
  - 2:1 AV block
- third-degree AV block.

*4. Is the PR segment elevated or depressed?*

If 'yes', consider:

- pericarditis
- atrial involvement in acute coronary syndrome.

## FURTHER READING

Epstein AE, DiMarco JP, Ellenbogen KA, *et al*. ACC/AHA/HRS 2008 Guidelines for device-based therapy of cardiac rhythm abnormalities. *J Am Coll Cardiol* 2008; **51**: e1–62.

Jim MH, Sio CW, Chan AOO, *et al*. Prognostic implications of PR-segment depression in inferior leads in acute inferior myocardial infarction. *Clin Cardiol* 2006; **29**: 363–368.

Keating L, Morris FP, Brady WJ. Electrocardiographic features of Wolff-Parkinson-White syndrome. *Emerg Med J* 2003; **20**: 491-493.

The Task Force for Cardiac Pacing and Cardiac Resynchronization Therapy of the European Society of Cardiology. Guidelines for cardiac pacing and cardiac resynchronization therapy. *Eur Heart J* 2007; **28**: 2256–2295.

After measuring the PR interval, go on to examine the QRS complex in each lead. Begin by looking for Q waves. A Q wave is present whenever the first deflection of the QRS complex points downwards (Fig. 13.1).

As you examine the QRS complex in each lead for the Q wave, the question to ask is:

● Are there any 'pathological' Q waves?

In this chapter we will help you to answer this question and to interpret any abnormality you may find.

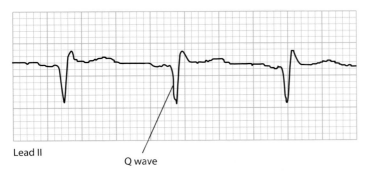

Lead II

Q wave

**Figure 13.1** The Q wave.

Key point:     ● A Q wave is present when the first QRS deflection is downwards.

## ARE THERE ANY 'PATHOLOGICAL' Q WAVES?

If Q waves are present, begin by asking: Could these be normal?

Q waves are usually absent from *most* of the leads of a normal ECG. However, *small* Q waves (often referred to as q waves) are normal in leads that look at the heart from the left: I, II, aVL, $V_5$ and $V_6$. They result from septal depolarization, which normally occurs from left to right, and hence are called 'septal' Q waves (Fig. 13.2).

A small Q wave may be normal in lead III, and is often associated with an inverted T wave (Fig. 13.3). Both may disappear on deep inspiration. Q waves are also normal in lead aVR.

Q waves in other leads are likely to be abnormal or 'pathological', particularly if they are:

● >2 small squares deep, or
● >25 per cent of the height of the following R wave in depth, and/or
● >1 small square wide.

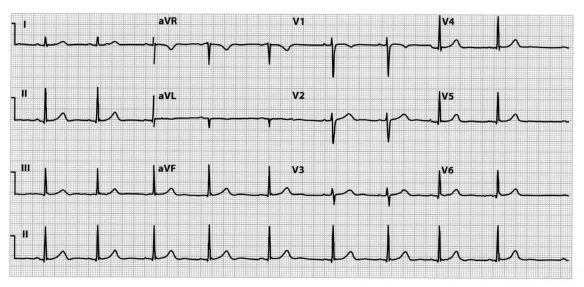

**Figure 13.2** Septal Q waves.

Key point:    • Small Q waves are seen in leads I, II, aVL, V$_5$ and V$_6$.

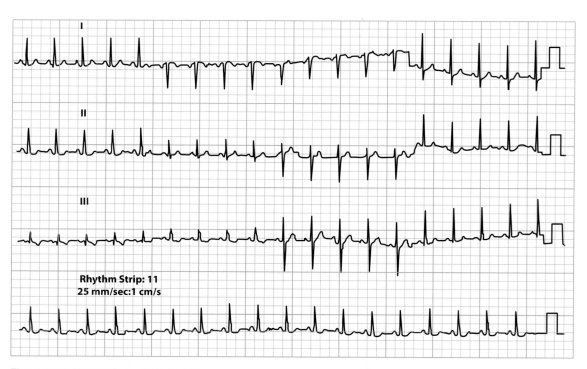

**Figure 13.3** Normal Q waves in lead III.

Key point:    • There are narrow Q waves in lead III, with inverted T waves.

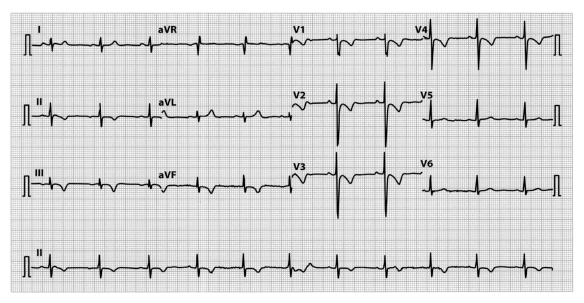

**Figure 13.4** Pulmonary embolism.

Key points:
- There is an $S_I Q_{III} T_{III}$ pattern.
- Note also the T wave inversion in leads $V_1$–$V_4$.
- The patient was taking beta-blockers, and so the usual sinus tachycardia was absent in this case.

If wide or deep Q waves (i.e. exceeding the above criteria) are present, consider:

- ST segment elevation myocardial infarction
- left ventricular hypertrophy
- Wolff–Parkinson–White syndrome
- bundle branch block.

Myocardial infarction, left ventricular hypertrophy and Wolff–Parkinson–White syndrome are discussed below. The bundle branch blocks are covered in detail in Chapters 9 and 14.

An abnormal Q wave (in lead III) is also a feature of:

- pulmonary embolism.

It is part of the 'classic' $S_I Q_{III} T_{III}$ pattern that is often quoted, although rarely seen (Fig. 13.4). However, the $Q_{III}$ rarely satisfies the 'pathological' Q wave criteria. The most frequent finding in pulmonary embolism is a tachycardia.

## ST segment elevation myocardial infarction

Q waves start to appear within a few hours of the onset of ST segment elevation myocardial infarction and in 90 per cent of cases become permanent. The presence of Q waves alone therefore gives no clue about the timing of the infarction. As with the other ECG changes in myocardial infarction, the location of the infarct can be determined from an analysis of the ECG leads (see Table 15.2, p. 162).

Figure 13.5 shows an ECG recorded on day 2 after an anterior ST segment elevation myocardial infarction. Q waves have developed in leads $V_1$–$V_3$.

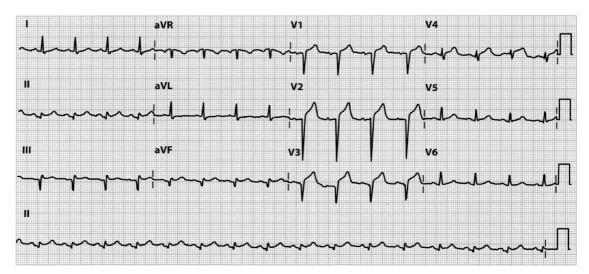

**Figure 13.5** Anteroseptal ST segment elevation myocardial infarction (day 2).

Key point:    • Q waves are seen in leads V₁–V₃, with residual ST segment elevation.

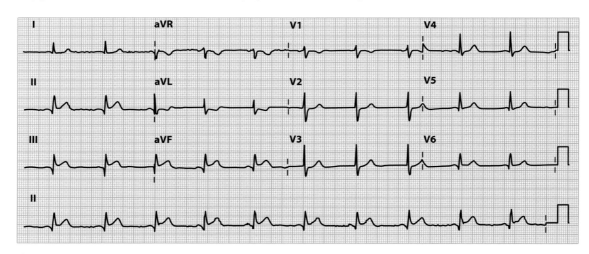

**Figure 13.6** Inferior myocardial infarction (after one year).

Key point:    • Q waves are present in leads II, III and aVF.

Figure 13.6 is from a patient who had an inferior myocardial infarction a year previously. Abnormal Q waves are seen in leads II, III and aVF.

The diagnosis of acute myocardial infarction is usually apparent from the presenting symptoms (chest pain, nausea and sweating) and ECG changes that are present, and can be confirmed by serial cardiac marker measurements. The management of acute myocardial infarction is discussed in detail in Chapter 15.

**ACT QUICKLY**

Acute coronary syndromes are a medical emergency. Prompt diagnosis and treatment are essential.

**13 The Q wave**

> **WHY DO Q WAVES APPEAR IN MYOCARDIAL INFARCTION?**
>
> Q waves develop in myocardial infarction following the necrosis (death) of an area of myocardium. The leads over the necrosed region can no longer record electrical activity in that area, and so they look 'through' it to record ventricular depolarization from 'within' the ventricular cavity rather than from outside.
>
> Because each wave of depolarization flows from the inner surface of the heart to the outer, a lead recording the depolarization from a viewpoint 'within' the ventricle would 'see' the electrical activity flowing away from it; hence, the negative deflection on the ECG – the Q wave.

When Q waves are found 'incidentally' on an ECG recorded for other reasons, a thorough review of the patient's history is necessary. Ask about:

- previous documented myocardial infarction
- previous symptoms suggestive of myocardial infarction
- symptoms of recent myocardial ischaemia.

However, bear in mind that approximately 20 per cent of myocardial infarctions are painless or 'silent'. If you remain uncertain about the importance of abnormal Q waves, and are suspicious about a previous myocardial infarction, there are many investigations that can help:

- echocardiography
- cardiac magnetic resonance imaging
- nuclear myocardial perfusion scan
- coronary angiography.

A cardiologist will be able to advise you on which of these tests, if any, are appropriate.

## Left ventricular hypertrophy

At the start of this chapter, we said that small ('septal') Q waves can be a normal finding and result from depolarization of the interventricular septum. If the septum hypertrophies, its muscle mass (and hence the amount of electricity generated by depolarization) increases, and the Q waves become deeper.

Left ventricular hypertrophy often involves the septum, and so deep Q waves are often seen in leads looking at the left and inferior surfaces of the heart.

Left ventricular hypertrophy is discussed more fully in Chapter 14.

## Wolff–Parkinson–White syndrome

The delta waves seen when there is a Wolff–Parkinson–White pattern on the ECG, indicating ventricular pre-excitation, can be negative in some leads (depending on the location of the accessory pathway). As such, these negative delta waves can be mistaken for Q waves, particularly when they are seen inferiorly (Fig. 13.7). This can lead to an incorrect diagnosis of myocardial infarction ('pseudo-infarction').

Ventricular pre-excitation and the Wolff–Parkinson–White syndrome are discussed more fully in Chapters 7 and 12.

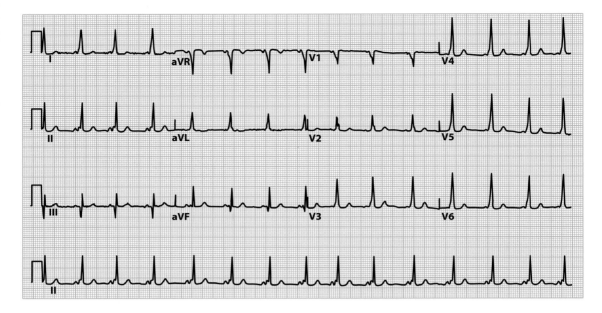

**Figure 13.7** Wolff–Parkinson–White pattern (type B).

Key point:      • There are negative delta waves in leads III and aVF, simulating the Q waves of an old inferior myocardial infarction.

---

## SUMMARY

To assess the Q wave, ask the following question:

*Are there any 'pathological' Q waves?*

If 'yes', consider:

- ST segment elevation myocardial infarction
- left ventricular hypertrophy
- Wolff–Parkinson–White syndrome
- bundle branch block.

Also:

- pulmonary embolism (although rarely 'pathological').

## FURTHER READING

Horan LG, Flowers NC, Johnson JC. Significance of the diagnostic Q wave of myocardial infarction. *Circulation* 1971; **43**: 428–436.

13 The Q wave

# CHAPTER 14

# The QRS complex

Normal QRS complexes have a different appearance in each of the 12 ECG leads (Fig. 14.1).

When reviewing an ECG, look carefully at the size and shape of the QRS complexes in each lead and ask yourself the following four questions:

- Are any R or S waves too big?
- Are the QRS complexes too small?
- Are any QRS complexes too wide?
- Are any QRS complexes an abnormal shape?

In this chapter, we will help you to answer these questions and to interpret any abnormalities you may find.

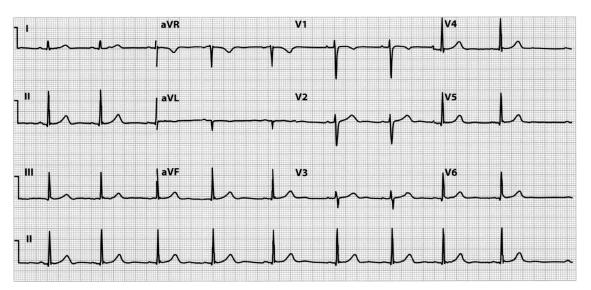

**Figure 14.1** Normal 12-lead ECG.

Key point:  • The size of the normal QRS complex varies from lead to lead.

## ARE ANY R OR S WAVES TOO BIG?

The height of the R wave and depth of the S wave vary from lead to lead in the normal ECG (as Fig. 14.1 shows). As a rule, in the normal ECG:

- the R wave *increases* in height from lead $V_1$ to $V_5$
- the R wave is *smaller* than the S wave in leads $V_1$ and $V_2$
- the R wave is *bigger* than the S wave in leads $V_5$ and $V_6$

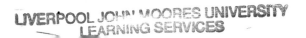

- the tallest R wave does not exceed 25 mm in height
- the deepest S wave does not exceed 25 mm in depth.

Always look carefully at the R and S waves in each lead, and check whether they conform to these criteria. If not, first of all consider:

- incorrect ECG calibration (should be 1 mV = 10 mm).

If the calibration is correct, consider whether your patient has one of the following:

- left ventricular hypertrophy
- right ventricular hypertrophy
- posterior myocardial infarction
- Wolff–Parkinson–White syndrome
- dextrocardia.

Each of these conditions is discussed below.

If the QRS complex is also abnormally wide, think of:

- bundle branch block (discussed later in this chapter).

## Left ventricular hypertrophy

Hypertrophy of the left ventricle causes tall R waves in the leads that 'look at' the left ventricle – I, aVL, $V_5$ and $V_6$ – and the reciprocal ('mirror image') change of deep S waves in leads that 'look at' the right ventricle – $V_1$ and $V_2$ (Fig. 14.2).

There are many criteria for the ECG diagnosis of left ventricular hypertrophy, with varying sensitivity and specificity. Generally, the diagnostic criteria are quite specific (if the criteria are present, the likelihood of the patient having left ventricular hypertrophy is >90 per cent), but not sensitive (the criteria will fail to detect 40–80 per cent of patients with left ventricular hypertrophy). The diagnostic criteria include:

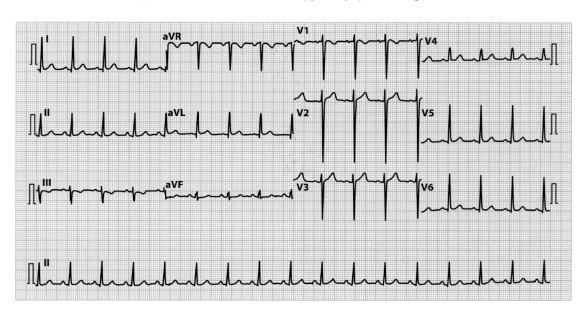

**Figure 14.2** Left ventricular hypertrophy.

Key point:    • Tall R waves in leads I, aVL, $V_5$ and $V_6$, with deep S waves in leads $V_1$, $V_2$ and $V_3$.

14 The QRS complex

- In the limb leads:
    - R wave >11 mm in lead aVL
    - R wave >20 mm in lead aVF
    - S wave >14 mm in lead aVR
    - sum of R wave in lead I and S wave in lead III >25 mm.
- In the chest leads:
    - R wave of ≥25 mm in the left chest leads
    - S wave of ≥25 mm in the right chest leads
    - sum of S wave in lead $V_1$ and R wave in lead $V_5$ or $V_6$ >35 mm (Sokolow–Lyon criterion)
    - sum of tallest R wave and deepest S wave in the chest leads >45 mm.

The **Cornell criteria** involve measuring the S wave in lead $V_3$ and the R wave in lead aVL. Left ventricular hypertrophy is indicated by a sum of >28 mm in men and >20 mm in women.

The **Romhilt–Estes scoring system** allocates points for the presence of certain criteria. A score of 5 indicates left ventricular hypertrophy and a score of 4 indicates probable left ventricular hypertrophy. Points are allocated as follows:

- 3 points – for (a) R or S wave in limb leads of ≥20 mm, (b) S wave in right chest leads of ≥25 mm, or (c) R wave in left chest leads of ≥25 mm
- 3 points – for ST segment and T wave changes ('typical strain') in a patient not taking digitalis (1 point with digitalis)
- 3 points – for P-terminal force in $V_1$ >1 mm deep with a duration >0.04 s
- 2 points – for left axis deviation (beyond –15°)
- 1 point – for QRS complex duration >0.09 s
- 1 point – for intrinsicoid deflection (the interval from the start of the QRS complex to the peak of the R wave) in $V_5$ or $V_6$ >0.05 s.

If there is evidence of left ventricular hypertrophy on the ECG, look also for evidence of 'strain':

- ST segment depression
- T wave inversion.

(See Fig. 15.17 for an example of left ventricular hypertrophy with 'strain'.)

Echocardiography is diagnostic for left ventricular hypertrophy. The treatment is usually that of the cause (Table 14.1).

Table 14.1 Causes of left ventricular hypertrophy

- Hypertension
- Aortic stenosis
- Coarctation of the aorta
- Hypertrophic cardiomyopathy

## Right ventricular hypertrophy

Right ventricular hypertrophy causes a 'dominant' R wave (i.e. bigger than the S wave) in the leads that 'look at' the right ventricle, particularly $V_1$ (Fig. 14.3).

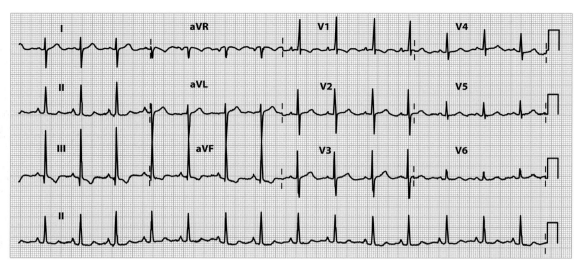

**Figure 14.3** Right ventricular hypertrophy.

Key point:   • There is a dominant R wave in lead V₁, together with right axis deviation.

---

**Table 14.2** Causes of right ventricular hypertrophy

- Pulmonary hypertension
- Pulmonary stenosis
- Pulmonary embolism
- Chronic pulmonary disease (cor pulmonale)
- Tetralogy of Fallot
- Arrhythmogenic right ventricular cardiomyopathy

---

Right ventricular hypertrophy is also associated with:

- right axis deviation (see Chapter 10)
- deep S waves in leads $V_5$ and $V_6$
- right bundle branch block (RBBB).

and, if 'strain' is present:

- ST segment depression
- T wave inversion.

If you suspect right ventricular hypertrophy, look for an underlying cause (Table 14.2). The treatment of right ventricular hypertrophy is that of the underlying cause.

## Posterior myocardial infarction

Posterior ST segment elevation myocardial infarction is one of the few causes of a 'dominant' R wave in lead $V_1$ (Table 14.3).

Infarction of the posterior wall of the left ventricle leads to reciprocal changes when viewed from the perspective of the anterior chest leads. Thus, the usual appearances of pathological Q waves, ST segment elevation and inverted T waves will appear as

---

**Table 14.3** Causes of a 'dominant' R wave in lead $V_1$

- Right ventricular hypertrophy
- Posterior myocardial infarction
- Wolff–Parkinson–White syndrome (left-sided accessory pathway)

---

*14 The QRS complex*

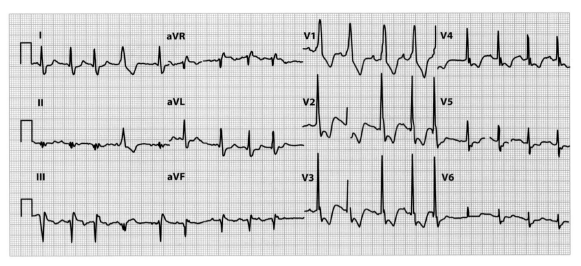

**Figure 14.4** Posterior myocardial infarction.

Key point:     • There is a dominant R wave in lead $V_1$, with ST segment depression in the anteroseptal chest leads.

*R waves*, ST segment *depression* and *upright*, *tall* T waves when viewed from leads $V_1$–$V_3$ (Fig. 14.4).

The management of acute myocardial infarction is discussed in detail in Chapter 15.

 **ACT QUICKLY**

> Acute myocardial infarction is a medical emergency. Prompt diagnosis and treatment are essential.

## Wolff–Parkinson–White syndrome

If you see a dominant R wave in leads $V_1$–$V_3$ in the presence of a short PR interval, think of Wolff–Parkinson–White syndrome (Fig. 14.5). Patients with Wolff–Parkinson–White syndrome have an accessory pathway (the bundle of Kent) that bypasses the atrioventricular node and bundle of His to connect the atria directly to the ventricles.

The position of the accessory pathway can be accurately localized only with electrophysiological studies. Generally, however, a dominant R wave in leads $V_1$–$V_3$ indicates a left-sided accessory pathway, whereas a dominant S wave in leads $V_1$–$V_3$ indicates a right-sided accessory pathway.

The management of Wolff–Parkinson–White syndrome is discussed in Chapter 7.

## Dextrocardia

In dextrocardia, the heart lies on the right side of the chest instead of the left. The ECG does not show the normal progressive increase in R wave height across the chest leads; instead, the QRS complexes decrease in height across them (Fig. 14.6). In addition, the P wave is inverted in lead I and there is right axis deviation. **Right-sided chest leads** will show the pattern normally seen on the left (Fig. 14.7).

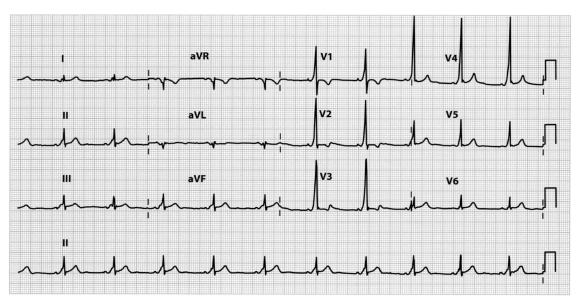

**Figure 14.5** Wolff–Parkinson–White pattern (Type A).

Key point:    • There is a dominant R wave in lead V₁, together with a short PR interval and delta wave.

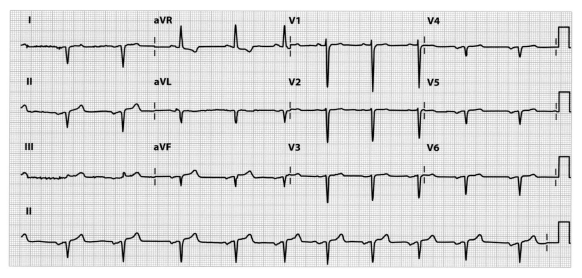

**Figure 14.6** Dextrocardia.

Key point:    • There is a decrease in R wave height across chest leads.

If you suspect dextrocardia, check the location of the patient's apex beat. A chest radiograph is diagnostic. No specific treatment is required for dextrocardia, but ensure the condition is highlighted in the patient's notes and check for any associated syndromes (e.g. Kartagener's syndrome – dextrocardia, bronchiectasis and sinusitis).

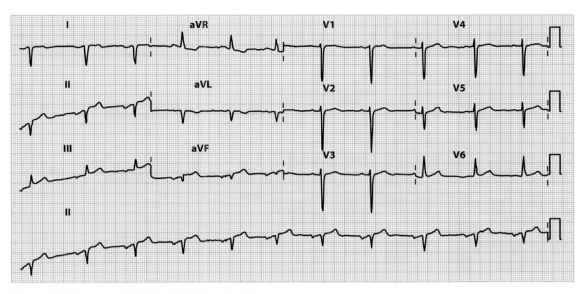

**Figure 14.7** Dextrocardia (right-sided chest leads).

Key point:    • Placing the chest electrodes in a mirror-image configuration across the right chest 'normalizes' the chest leads in dextrocardia.

## ARE THE QRS COMPLEXES TOO SMALL?

Small QRS complexes indicate that relatively little of the voltage generated by ventricular depolarization is reaching the ECG electrodes. Although criteria exist for the normal upper limit of QRS complex size, there are no similar guidelines for the lower limit of QRS size.

Small QRS complexes may simply reflect a variant of normal. However, always check for:

• incorrect ECG calibration (should be 1 mV = 10 mm).

Also check whether the patient has:

• obesity
• emphysema.

Both of these conditions increase the distance between the heart and the chest electrodes.

However, if the QRS complexes appear small, and particularly if they have changed in relation to earlier ECG recordings, always consider the possibility of:

• pericardial effusion.

This is discussed below.

### Pericardial effusion

Pericardial effusion reduces the voltage of the QRS complexes (Fig. 14.8). Pericardial effusion can also cause electrical alternans, in which the height of the R waves and/or T waves alternates from beat to beat (Fig. 14.9).

Pericardial effusion may be asymptomatic when small. Larger effusions cause breathlessness and, ultimately, cardiac tamponade. The presence of Beck's triad indicates major cardiac compromise:

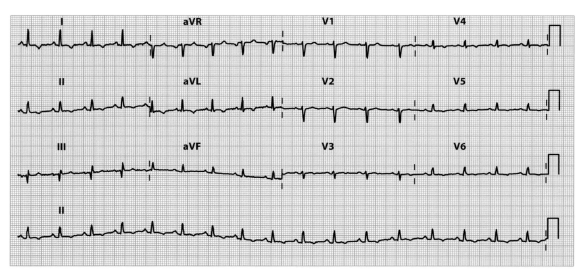

**Figure 14.8** Pericardial effusion.

Key point:    • There are relatively small QRS complexes because the current reaching the ECG electrodes is reduced by the effusion.

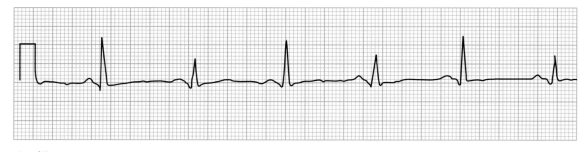

Lead II

**Figure 14.9** Electrical alternans in pericardial effusion.

Key point:    • There is a beat-to-beat variation in R wave height.

- low blood pressure
- elevated jugular venous pressure
- impalpable apex beat.

In addition, the heart sounds are soft and there may be pulsus paradoxus (a marked fall in blood pressure on inspiration). The combination of small QRS complexes, electrical alternans and a tachycardia is a highly specific, but insensitive, indicator of a pericardial tamponade.

In a patient with a pericardial effusion, the chest radiograph may show a large globular heart but with no distension of the pulmonary veins. The echocardiogram is diagnostic.

Obtain the advice of a cardiologist immediately, particularly if the effusion is causing haemodynamic impairment. Urgent pericardial aspiration is required if the signs of tamponade are present, but should only be undertaken by, or under the guidance of, someone experienced in the procedure.

14 The QRS complex

**ACT QUICKLY**

Cardiac tamponade is a medical emergency. Prompt diagnosis and treatment are essential.

## ARE ANY QRS COMPLEXES TOO WIDE?

The QRS complex corresponds to depolarization of the ventricles, and this normally takes no longer than 0.12 s from start to finish. Thus, the width of a normal QRS complex is no greater than 3 small squares on the ECG.

Widening of the QRS complex is seen if conduction through the ventricles is slower than normal, and this usually means that depolarization has taken an abnormal route through the ventricles, as happens in:

- bundle branch block
- ventricular rhythms.

These conditions are discussed below.

Widening of the QRS complex can also result from:

- hyperkalaemia.

Hyperkalaemia is discussed on page 180.

### Bundle branch block

After leaving the bundle of His, the conduction fibres divide into two pathways as they pass through the interventricular septum – the left and right bundle branches, which supply the left and right ventricles, respectively.

A block of either of the bundle branches delays the electrical activation of its ventricle, which must instead be depolarized *indirectly* via the other bundle branch. This prolongs the process of ventricular depolarization, and so the QRS complex is wider than 3 small squares. In addition, the shape of the QRS complex is distorted because of the abnormal pathway of depolarization.

The causes and mechanisms of left bundle branch block (LBBB, Fig. 14.10) and right bundle branch block (RBBB, Fig. 14.11) are both discussed in detail in Chapter 9.

The presence of LBBB is almost invariably an indication of underlying pathology (Table 9.2), and the patient should be assessed accordingly. New-onset LBBB can be the presenting ECG feature of acute myocardial infarction, and is an indication for urgent reperfusion. The presence of LBBB greatly limits further interpretation of the ECG beyond the QRS complex.

CABRERA'S SIGN

The presence of LBBB makes interpretation of the ECG beyond the QRS complex extremely challenging. As a result, it can be very difficult to recognize previous myocardial infarction in a patient with pre-existing LBBB. However, Cabrera's sign can help. This is the presence of a notch 40 msec into the ascending portion of the S wave in leads $V_3$ and $V_4$ (Fig. 14.12). Cabrera's sign has a high specificity (but a poor sensitivity) for previous myocardial infarction in LBBB.

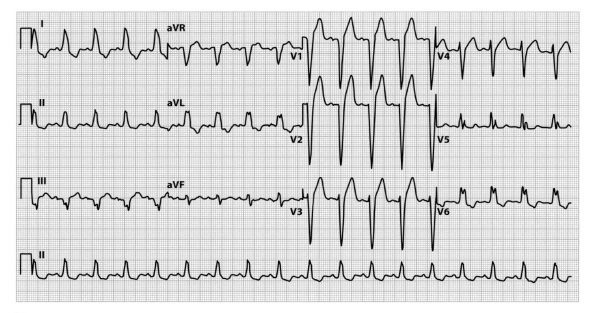

**Figure 14.10** Left bundle branch block.

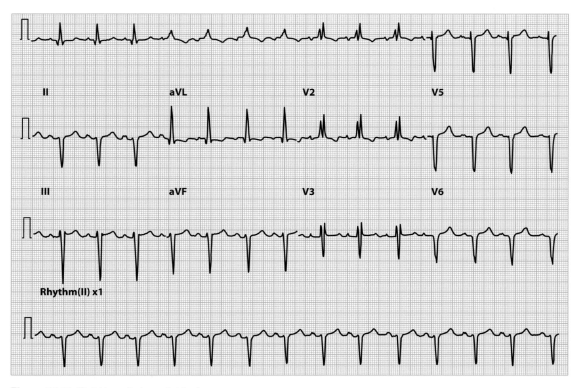

**Figure 14.11** Right bundle branch block.

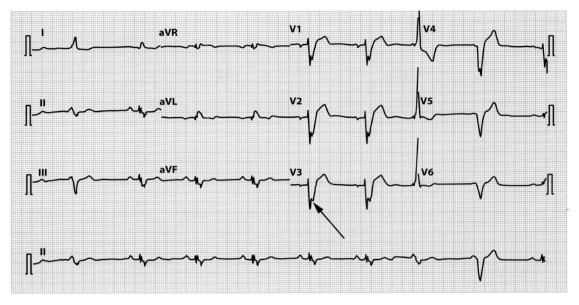

**Figure 14.12** Cabrera's sign.

Key point:
- There is a notch 40 ms into the ascending portion of the S wave in lead $V_3$ (arrowed), indicative of previous myocardial infarction in a patient with LBBB.

---

## SGARBOSSA CRITERIA

The Sgarbossa criteria are a scoring system for identifying acute myocardial infarction in the presence of LBBB (or a paced rhythm) on the ECG. There are three criteria:

- ST segment elevation ≥1 mm and concordant with QRS complex (5 points)
- ST segment depression ≥1 mm in lead $V_1$, $V_2$, or $V_3$ (3 points)
- ST segment elevation ≥5 mm and discordant with QRS complex (2 points)

A score of ≥3 points has a high specificity (but low sensitivity) for acute myocardial infarction in the setting of LBBB.

In contrast with LBBB, RBBB is a relatively common finding in otherwise normal hearts. However, it too can result from underlying disease (Table 9.3) and should be investigated according to the clinical presentation.

Bundle branch block (particularly RBBB) can also occur at fast heart rates. This is not uncommonly seen during supraventricular tachycardia (SVT), and the resultant broad complexes can lead to an incorrect diagnosis of ventricular tachycardia (VT) by the unwary. For help in distinguishing between VT and SVT, see page 86.

Both LBBB and RBBB are asymptomatic in themselves, and do not require treatment in their own right. Even so, they should prompt you to look for an underlying cause that is appropriate to the patient's presentation.

## Ventricular rhythms

When depolarization is initiated from within the ventricular muscle itself, the wave of electrical activity has to spread from myocyte to myocyte rather than using the more rapid Purkinje network. This prolongs the process of ventricular depolarization and thus widens the QRS complex (Fig. 8.7).

For more information about ventricular rhythms, and help with their identification, see Chapter 8.

## ARE ANY QRS COMPLEXES AN ABNORMAL SHAPE?

Most of the causes of an abnormally shaped QRS complex have been discussed earlier in this chapter. However, occasionally you will encounter QRS complexes that just appear unusual, without fitting any of the specific criteria mentioned above.

You may see complexes which appear 'slurred', or have an abnormal 'notch', without necessarily being abnormally tall, small or wide. If this is the case, consider the following possible causes:

- incomplete bundle branch block
- fascicular block
- Wolff–Parkinson–White syndrome.

Further information on each of these can be found below.

### Incomplete bundle branch block

Bundle branch block is discussed earlier in this chapter. Sometimes, however, conduction down a bundle branch can be *delayed* without being blocked entirely. When this happens, the QRS complex develops an abnormal shape but the complex remains less than 3 small squares wide. This is called incomplete (or partial) bundle branch block, and can affect either the left or the right bundle branches (Figs. 14.13 and 14.14).

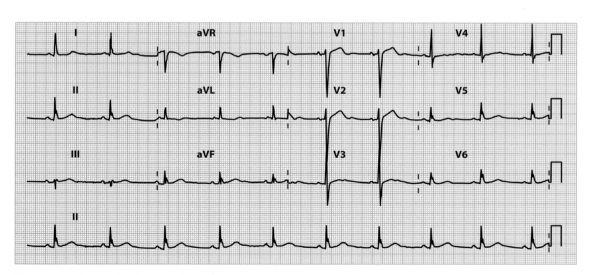

**Figure 14.13** Incomplete left bundle branch block.

Key point:    • There is a left bundle branch block morphology, but with a normal QRS complex duration.

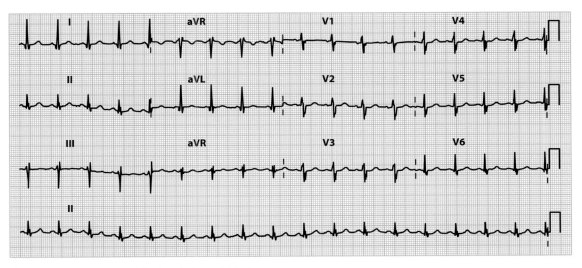

**Figure 14.14** Incomplete right bundle branch block.

Key point:    • There is a right bundle branch block morphology, but with a normal QRS complex duration.

The causes of incomplete bundle branch block are the same as those of complete bundle branch block, discussed earlier in this chapter.

## Fascicular block

Block of one of the two fascicles of the left bundle causes either left or right axis deviation. The consequent delay to conduction may also lead to slurring or notching of the QRS complex. How to identify which fascicle is affected, and manage the patient subsequently, is discussed in Chapter 10.

## Wolff–Parkinson–White syndrome

Patients with Wolff–Parkinson–White syndrome characteristically exhibit a delta wave that slurs the upstroke of the QRS complex (Fig. 7.15). This diagnosis should be suspected if, in addition, the PR interval is abnormally short. For more information on the diagnosis and management of Wolff–Parkinson–White syndrome, see Chapter 7.

---

### SUMMARY

To assess the QRS complex, ask the following questions:

*1. Are any R or S waves too big?*

If 'yes', consider:

- incorrect ECG calibration
- left ventricular hypertrophy
- right ventricular hypertrophy
- posterior myocardial infarction
- Wolff–Parkinson–White syndrome (left-sided accessory pathway)
- dextrocardia.

*(Continued)*

*(Continued)*

Also:

- bundle branch block.

*2. Are the QRS complexes too small?*

If 'yes', consider:

- incorrect ECG calibration
- obesity
- emphysema
- pericardial effusion.

*3. Are any QRS complexes too wide?*

If 'yes', consider:

- bundle branch block
- ventricular rhythms.

Also:

- hyperkalaemia.

*4. Are any QRS complexes an abnormal shape?*

If 'yes', consider:

- incomplete bundle branch block
- fascicular block
- Wolff–Parkinson–White syndrome.

## FURTHER READING

Bauml MA, Underwood DA. Left ventricular hypertrophy: an overlooked cardiovascular risk factor. *Cleveland Clinic J Med* 2010; **77**: 381–387.

Francia P, Balla C, Paneni F, *et al*. Left bundle-branch block – pathophysiology, prognosis, and clinical management. *Clin Cardiol* 2007; **30**: 110–115.

Hancock EW, Deal BJ, Mirvis DM, *et al*. AHA/ACCF/HRS recommendations for the standardization and interpretation of the electrocardiogram: Part V: Electrocardiogram changes associated with cardiac chamber hypertrophy. *J Am Coll Cardiol* 2009; **53**: 992–1002.

Sgarbossa EB, Pinski SL, Barbagelata A, *et al*. Electrocardiographic diagnosis of evolving acute myocardial infarction in the presence of left bundle-branch block. *N Engl J Med* 1996; **334**: 481–487.

# CHAPTER 15

# The ST segment

The ST segment lies between the end of the S wave and the start of the T wave. Normally, the ST segment is isoelectric, meaning that it lies at the same level as the ECG's baseline, the horizontal line between the end of the T wave and the start of the P wave (Fig. 15.1).

ST segments can be abnormal in one of three ways, so the questions you need to ask about the ST segments when you review them are:

- Are the ST segments elevated?
- Are the ST segments depressed?
- Are J waves present?

In this chapter, we will help you to answer these questions, and guide you about what to do next if you find an abnormality.

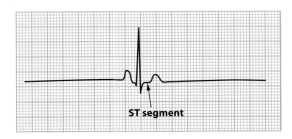

**ST segment**

**Figure 15.1** The ST segment.

Key point:  • Normally, the ST segment is isoelectric.

## ARE THE ST SEGMENTS ELEVATED?

Look carefully at the ST segment in each lead to see if it is isoelectric. If it is raised above this level, the ST segment is elevated.

ST segment elevation should never be ignored, as it often indicates a serious problem that warrants urgent attention. If you see ST segment elevation in any lead, consider the following possible diagnoses:

- ST segment elevation myocardial infarction
- left ventricular aneurysm
- Prinzmetal's (vasospastic) angina
- pericarditis
- left bundle branch block
- Brugada syndrome
- high take-off (diagnose this only if you have excluded all other causes).

**Table 15.1** Risk factors for cardiovascular disease

Modifiable:
- Cigarette smoking
- Hypertension
- Diabetes mellitus
- Dyslipidaemia
- Overweight and obesity
- Physical inactivity

Non-modifiable:
- Age
- Male sex
- Family history

Therefore, ST segment elevation can represent anything from a potentially life-threatening condition to a normal variant, making it particularly important to identify the cause. To help you in this task, we describe each of these conditions (together with example ECGs) below.

CHEST PAIN SUGGESTIVE OF ACUTE CORONARY SYNDROME

The key symptoms of acute coronary syndrome are:

- tight, central chest pain (usually severe, and longer lasting, than that of angina)
- breathlessness
- nausea and vomiting
- sweating ('diaphoresis').

Ask about a history of previous angina or myocardial infarction, or any other form of vascular disease (stroke/TIA or peripheral vascular disease) and assess cardiovascular risk factors (Table 15.1). An urgent ECG is mandatory in patients presenting with chest pain suggestive of acute coronary syndrome.

## ST segment elevation myocardial infarction

Patients presenting with acute coronary syndromes are ultimately divided into three categories:

- ST segment elevation myocardial infarction (STEMI)
- non-ST segment elevation myocardial infarction (NSTEMI)
- unstable angina.

All three groups of patients present with similar symptoms – ischaemic chest pain (tight, central), often with breathlessness, sweating, nausea and vomiting – and the initial categorization is made on the basis of the presenting ECG (Fig. 15.2). If there is ST segment elevation, the patient is managed as STEMI. If the ST segment is depressed, or there is T wave inversion, or the ECG is normal, then the working diagnosis is either NSTEMI or unstable angina (and the distinction between these is made later when the troponin results are available).

This section is chiefly concerned with STEMI. More information about NSTEMI can be found on page 174.

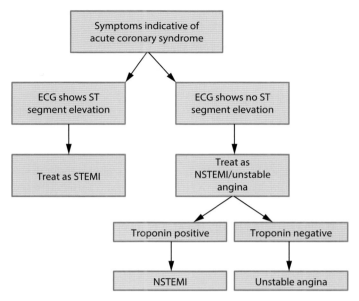

**Figure 15.2** Acute coronary syndromes.

Key point:   • The diagnostic category of acute coronary syndrome is based upon the presenting symptoms, the ECG findings and whether there has been myocyte necrosis (as evidenced by the troponin results).

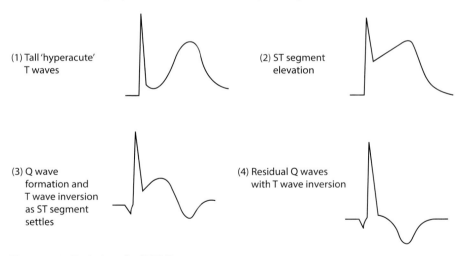

**Figure 15.3** Evolution of a STEMI.

Key points:   • Tall 'hyperacute' T waves may be the earliest finding, rapidly followed by ST segment elevation.
• As the ST segment settles, the T wave inverts and Q waves form.
• The Q waves and inverted T waves may persist indefinitely.

In STEMI, the ECG changes gradually 'evolve' in the sequence shown in Figure 15.3. The earliest change is ST segment elevation accompanied, or even preceded, by tall 'hyperacute' T waves. Over the next few hours or days, Q waves appear, the ST segments return to normal and the T waves become inverted. It is usual for some permanent abnormality of the ECG to persist following STEMI – usually 'pathological' Q waves, although the T waves may remain inverted permanently too.

**Table 15.2** Localization of ST segment elevation acute myocardial infarction

| Leads containing ST segment elevation | Location of event |
|---|---|
| $V_1$–$V_4$ | Anterior |
| I, aVL, $V_5$–$V_6$ | Lateral |
| I, aVL, $V_1$–$V_6$ | Anterolateral |
| $V_1$–$V_3$ | Anteroseptal |
| II, III, aVF | Inferior |
| I, aVL, $V_5$–$V_6$, II, III, aVF | Inferolateral |

Do not forget that acute myocardial infarction can also present with the new onset of left bundle branch block on the ECG (Chapter 14), and patients presenting in this way are managed in the same way as those with ST segment elevation.

The ECG also allows you to identify the area of myocardium affected by STEMI, as the leads 'looking at' that area will be the ones in which abnormalities are seen (Table 15.2). Examples of ST segment elevation in different myocardial territories are shown in Figures 15.4–15.6.

---

**AORTIC DISSECTION**

Beware of missing a diagnosis of aortic dissection. This too can cause ST segment elevation (if the dissection involves the coronary arteries) and chest pain, but patients may also complain of a 'tearing' back pain with different blood pressure in each arm, and a chest radiograph will show mediastinal widening. The diagnosis can be confirmed by a CT aortogram.

---

Having diagnosed STEMI, waste no time in admitting the patient to a coronary care unit or other monitored area for treatment as indicated. This is discussed later in this section.

If you diagnose an inferior STEMI, go on to ask the question:

- Is the right ventricle involved?

To make the diagnosis, record another ECG, but this time use right-sided chest leads (Fig. 15.7). Look for ST segment elevation in lead $V_4R$ (Fig. 15.8). If present, there is a high likelihood of right ventricular involvement.

Patients with STEMI require:

- pain relief (an opioid intravenously and an anti-emetic)
- oxygen if hypoxic
- aspirin, 300 mg orally
- clopidogrel, 300 mg orally.

The main priority in STEMI is urgent primary percutaneous coronary intervention (PCI) or, if facilities for coronary angiography and primary PCI are unavailable, intravenous administration of a thrombolytic agent may be considered. Thrombolysis is indicated (unless contraindicated) in patients whose history suggests a myocardial infarction within the past 12 h and whose ECG shows:

- ST segment elevation consistent with infarction, or
- new left bundle branch block.

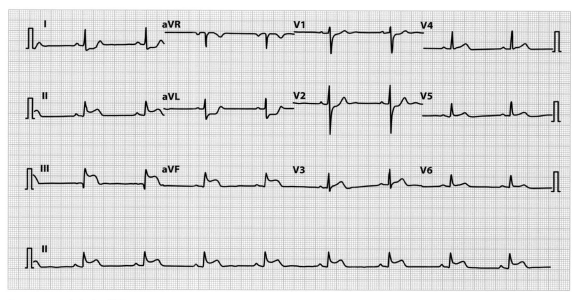

**Figure 15.4** Inferior STEMI.

Key point:   • There is ST segment elevation in leads II, III and aVF, with 'reciprocal' ST segment depression in leads I and aVL.

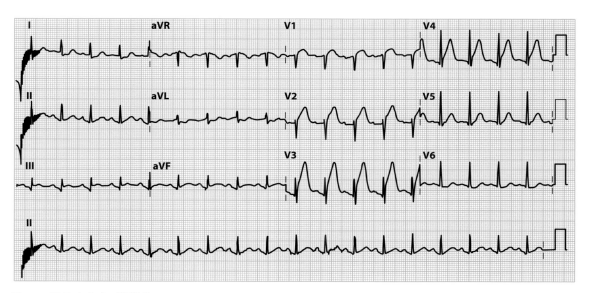

**Figure 15.5** Anterior STEMI.

Key point:   • There is ST segment elevation in leads $V_1$–$V_4$.

Following STEMI, patients should continue with:

- aspirin, 75 mg daily
- clopidogrel, 75 mg daily (short term)
- a beta blocker
- an angiotensin-converting enzyme inhibitor

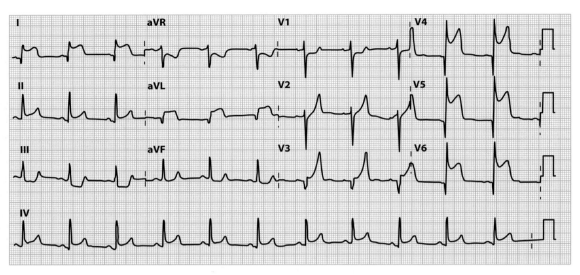

**Figure 15.6** Anterolateral STEMI.

Key point:    • There is ST segment elevation in leads $V_4$–$V_6$, I and aVL.

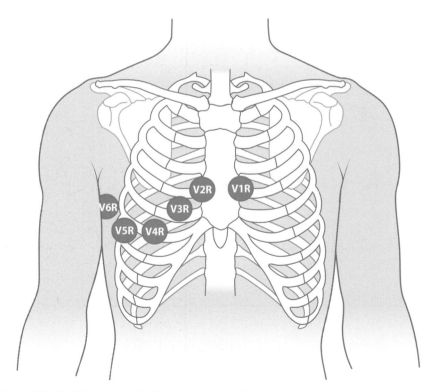

**Figure 15.7** Positioning of right-sided chest electrodes.

Key point:    • On the ECG, the chest leads should be labelled $V_1R$–$V_6R$ and the ECG itself should be clearly labelled 'right-sided leads'.

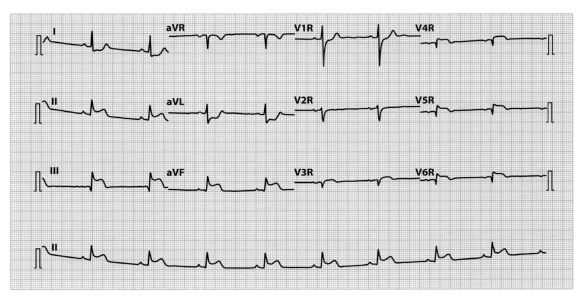

**Figure 15.8** Inferior STEMI with right ventricular involvement.

Key points:
- There is inferior ST segment elevation (leads II, III and aVF).
- ST segment elevation in lead $V_4R$ indicates right ventricular involvement.

---

WHY IS RIGHT VENTRICULAR INFARCTION IMPORTANT?

Patients with right ventricular infarction may develop the signs of right-sided heart failure (elevated jugular venous pressure and peripheral oedema). The left ventricle may be functioning normally, so the lungs are clear.

If these patients develop hypotension, it is usually because their left-sided filling pressure is too low (as the supply of blood from the damaged right ventricle is inadequate). Vasodilator drugs must be avoided. Intravenous fluids may be needed to maintain right ventricular output, thus ensuring sufficient blood is supplied to the left ventricle.

It may seem paradoxical to give intravenous fluids to patients who already appear to be in right heart failure, unless the reasons for doing so are understood. If haemodynamically compromised, these patients need fluid balance monitoring using a Swan–Ganz catheter, which measures right-sided and, indirectly, left-sided filling pressure. The risk of severe complications is high in these patients.

---

- prophylactic subcutaneous heparin until mobile
- a statin.

 **ACT QUICKLY**

Acute coronary syndrome is a medical emergency. Prompt diagnosis and treatment are essential.

## Left ventricular aneurysm

The development of a left ventricular aneurysm is a late complication of myocardial infarction, seen (to varying degrees) in about 10 per cent of survivors. The presence of an aneurysm can lead to persistent ST segment elevation in those chest leads that 'look at' the affected region (Fig. 15.9).

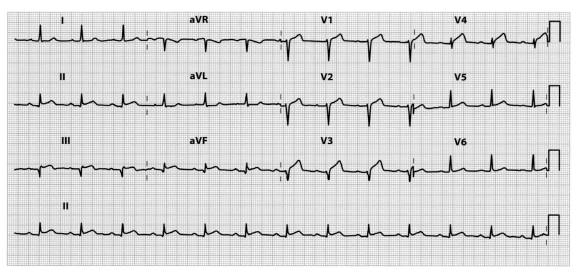

**Figure 15.9** Left ventricular aneurysm.

Key point:     • Persistent ST segment elevation in leads $V_1$–$V_4$ six months following an anterior STEMI.

Ask the patient about a history of previous myocardial infarction and assess the patient for symptoms and signs related to the aneurysm itself. Aneurysms, being non-contractile, can lead to left ventricular dysfunction and thrombus formation. They can also be a focus for arrhythmia generation. Presenting symptoms can result from:

- heart failure
- embolic events
- arrhythmias.

The clinical signs of a left ventricular aneurysm are a 'double impulse' on precordial palpation and a fourth heart sound on auscultation. A chest radiograph may reveal a bulge on the cardiac outline. The investigation of choice is echocardiography, which will reveal the site of the aneurysm and the presence of mural thrombus, as well as allowing assessment of overall left ventricular function.

Patients with left ventricular aneurysms may benefit from treatment for heart failure and use of anticoagulation and anti-arrhythmic drugs. Consideration may also be given to surgical removal of the aneurysm (aneurysmectomy) or even cardiac transplantation where appropriate. Specialist referral is therefore recommended.

**SEEK HELP**

A left ventricular aneurysm warrants specialist assessment. Obtain the advice of a cardiologist without delay.

## Prinzmetal's (vasospastic) angina

Prinzmetal's angina refers to reversible myocardial ischaemia that results from coronary artery spasm. Although it can occur with normal coronary arteries, in over 90 per cent of cases the spasm is superimposed on some degree of atherosclerosis. Although any artery can be affected, spasm most commonly occurs in the right coronary artery. During an episode of vasospasm, the patient develops ST segment elevation in the affected territory (Fig. 15.10).

15 The ST segment

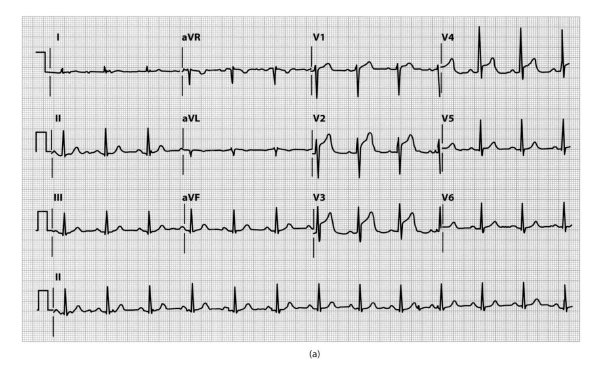

(a)

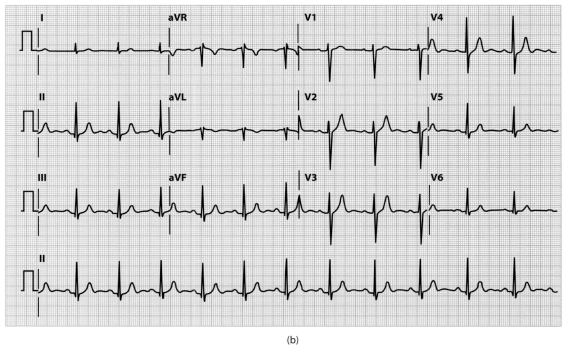

(b)

**Figure 15.10** Prinzmetal's (vasospastic) angina.

Key points:  • ECG (a) shows anterior ST segment elevation during episode of chest pain.
           • ECG (b) shows the ST segment elevation resolving as the chest pain settles.

Although the combination of chest pain and ST segment elevation often suggests STEMI, vasospastic angina is distinguished by the transient nature of the ST segment elevation. Unlike STEMI, the ECG changes of vasospastic angina resolve entirely when the episode of chest pain settles. Ask the patient about prior episodes of chest pain, which typically occur at rest and particularly overnight in vasospastic angina. Patients may also have a history of other vasospastic disorders, such as Raynaud's phenomenon.

The ST segment elevation of vasospastic angina may be accompanied by tall 'hyper-acute' T waves or, sometimes, T wave inversion. Transient intraventricular conduction defects, such as a bundle branch or fascicular block, can also occur. Treatment for vasospastic angina should include a calcium channel blocker and/or a nitrate. Vasospastic angina can worsen with use of beta blockers, because they block the vasodilatory effects of beta receptors while leaving vasoconstrictor alpha receptors unblocked.

## Pericarditis

The ST segment elevation of pericarditis (Fig. 15.11) has four characteristics that, while not pathognomonic, help to distinguish it from STEMI:

- The ST segment elevation is typically widespread, affecting all of those leads (anterolateral and inferior) that 'look at' the inflamed epicardium. Leads aVR and $V_1$ usually show reciprocal ST segment depression.
- The ST segment elevation is characteristically 'saddle shaped' (concave upward).
- T wave inversion occurs only after the ST segments have returned to baseline.
- Q waves do not develop.

The assessment of a patient with pericarditis should aim not only to confirm the diagnosis but also at establishing the cause (Table 15.3).

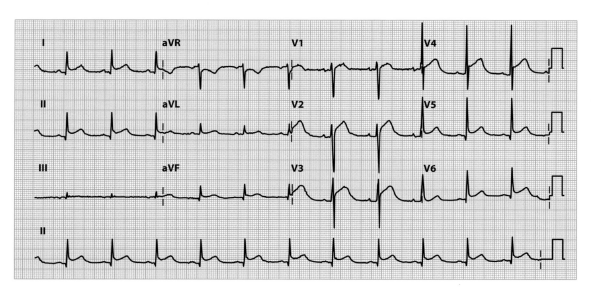

**Figure 15.11** Pericarditis.

Key point:    • Widespread 'saddle-shaped' ST segment elevation.

**Table 15.3** Causes of pericarditis

- Infectious
  - viral (e.g. coxsackie)
  - bacterial (e.g. tuberculosis, *Staphylococcus*)
  - fungal
  - parasitic
- Myocardial infarction (first few days)
- Dressler's syndrome (1 month or more post-myocardial infarction)
- Uraemia
- Malignancy
- Connective tissue disease
- Radiotherapy
- Traumatic
- Drug-induced

Pericarditis can also cause depression of the PR segment, which is thought to be caused by atrial involvement in the inflammatory process. PR segment depression is a specific ECG feature of pericarditis and may be seen in any leads except aVR and $V_1$ (where there may be PR segment elevation).

Clinically, the pain of pericarditis can usually be distinguished from that of myocardial infarction. Although both produce a retrosternal pain, the pain of pericarditis is sharp and pleuritic, exacerbated by inspiration and relieved by sitting forwards. A friction rub on auscultation is pathognomonic of pericarditis.

Direct treatment of the underlying cause should be carried out where possible. Anti-inflammatory agents (e.g. aspirin, indometacin) are often effective. Colchicine can be useful in treating relapsing pericarditis. Systemic corticosteroids can be considered in selected cases, although their role is controversial and they should not be considered without first obtaining specialist advice.

## Left bundle branch block

Persistent elevation of the ST segment is a normal feature of the right precordial leads ($V_1$–$V_3$) in left bundle branch block (LBBB, Fig. 15.12). In LBBB this is known as 'appropriate discordance' (see box). LBBB is discussed in more detail in Chapter 14.

### DIAGNOSING STEMI IN PATIENTS WITH LBBB

The abnormal pattern of ventricular depolarization in LBBB is followed by an abnormal pattern of repolarization. This manifests itself on the ECG by repolarization (ST segment and T wave) appearances that are discordant with the depolarization (QRS complex) appearances. In other words, where the QRS complex is negative, the following ST segment will be 'positive' (elevated) and the T wave will also be 'positive' (upright). This is known as 'appropriate discordance'.

One useful aspect of this concept is that the presence of *concordance* between the QRS complex and the subsequent ST segment and T wave in the setting of LBBB can be used as an indicator of myocardial ischaemia or infarction. This can be termed 'inappropriate concordance' and applies to ST segment elevation/upright T waves following a positive QRS complex, or ST segment depression/inverted T waves following a negative QRS complex (i.e. in leads $V_1$–$V_3$).

**Sgarbossa** (*see Further Reading*) has described criteria for diagnosing STEMI in the presence of LBBB:

*(Continued)*

(*Continued*)

- 5 points are scored if there is ST segment elevation ≥1 mm in at least one lead with a positive QRS complex
- 3 points are scored if there is ST segment depression ≥1 mm in leads $V_1$–$V_3$
- 2 points are scored if there is ≥5 mm ST segment elevation in leads with a negative QRS complex.

A score of 3 points or more has a 90% specificity (but a poor sensitivity) for the diagnosis of STEMI.

## Brugada syndrome

Brugada syndrome is a hereditary (autosomal dominant) condition caused by an abnormality of the cardiac sodium channel, and is characterized on the ECG by a right bundle branch block morphology and persistent ST segment elevation in leads $V_1$–$V_3$ (Fig. 15.13). Brugada syndrome predisposes the patient to syncope and sudden cardiac death secondary to ventricular arrhythmias. It is thought to be responsible for as many as 50 per cent of cases of sudden cardiac death with an 'apparently normal' heart.

Three different ECG patterns have been described in Brugada syndrome. All three have ST segment elevation (≥2 mm elevation of the J point), but vary in other ways:

- Type 1 has 'coved' ST segment elevation with inverted T waves. The terminal portion of the ST segment gradually descends until it meets the inverted T wave.
- Type 2 has saddle-shaped ST segment elevation with positive or biphasic T waves. The terminal portion of the ST segment is elevated by ≥1 mm.
- Type 3 has saddle-shaped ST segment elevation with positive T waves. The terminal portion of the ST segment is elevated by <1 mm.

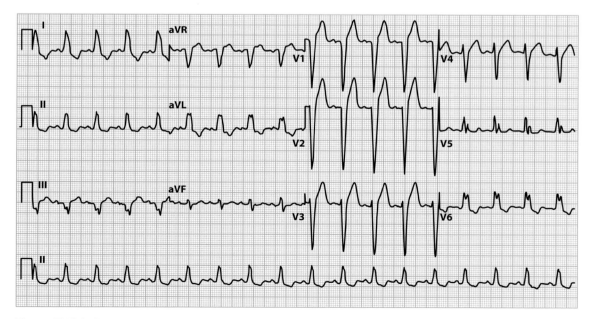

**Figure 15.12** Left bundle branch block.

Key point:    • ST segment elevation is a normal finding in leads with a negative QRS complex in LBBB.

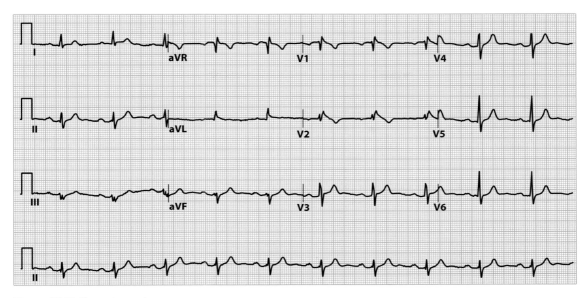

**Figure 15.13** Brugada syndrome.

Key points:
- This ECG was recorded during an ajmaline challenge.
- There is a right bundle branch block morphology with ST segment elevation and T wave inversion in leads V$_1$ and V$_2$.

Recording the 12-lead ECG with leads V$_1$ and V$_2$ in the second (rather than fourth) intercostal space has been reported to increase the diagnostic sensitivity of the ECG. Some patients require an intravenous challenge with a sodium channel blocking drug (such as flecainide or ajmaline) to unmask the ECG appearances. This is not helpful in those with a Type 1 ECG, but can help diagnostically in those with Type 2 or 3 ECG appearances. Such a test should only be performed by individuals trained and experienced in the technique.

**SEEK HELP**

Brugada syndrome can be challenging to diagnose, and poses a risk of life-threatening arrhythmias. Patients may benefit from implantation of a cardioverter defibrillator. Prompt referral to a cardiologist is important.

## High take-off

Elevation of the ST segment is sometimes seen in the anterior chest leads as a variant of normal, and is referred to as 'high take-off' or 'early repolarization'. A high take-off ST segment always follows an S wave and is not associated with reciprocal ST segment depression; compare its appearances in Figure 15.14 with the earlier ECGs in this chapter.

Whenever you suspect ST segment elevation to be just high take-off, always endeavour to find earlier ECGs for confirmation.

## ARE THE ST SEGMENTS DEPRESSED?

Again, look carefully at the ST segment in each lead to see if it is isoelectric (on the same level as the ECG's baseline). If it is below this level, the ST segment is depressed.

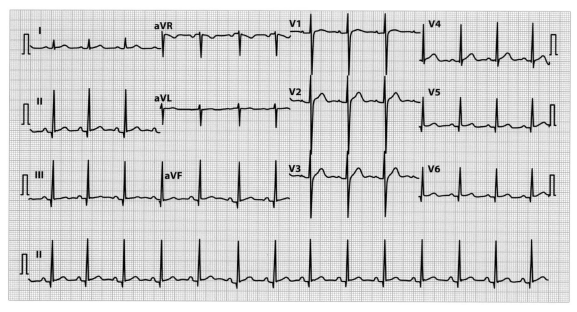

**Figure 15.14** High take-off.

Key point:    • ST segment elevation following an S wave, as seen in the chest leads $V_2$–$V_4$.

If ST segment depression is present, think of the following possible causes:

- myocardial ischaemia
- acute posterior myocardial infarction
- 'reciprocal' changes in ST segment elevation myocardial infarction
- drugs (e.g. digoxin)
- ventricular hypertrophy with 'strain'.

If any of these is a possibility, turn to the following pages for guidance on what to do next.

## Myocardial ischaemia

Unlike myocardial infarction, ischaemia is reversible and so the associated ECG abnormalities are seen only while the patient is experiencing an episode of pain. ST segment depression is the commonest abnormality associated with ischaemia and is usually 'horizontal' (cf. the 'reverse tick' with digoxin effect, p. 175).

Other changes seen in myocardial ischaemia include:

- T wave inversion (Chapter 16)
- T wave 'pseudonormalization' (Chapter 16).

Figure 15.15 shows the ECG of a patient with coronary artery disease during an episode of chest pain.

If myocardial ischaemia is a possibility in your patient, ask about prior episodes of angina and myocardial infarctions. Also ask about risk factors for coronary artery disease (see Table 15.1, p. 160). The characteristic features of stable angina are:

- central chest tightness/heaviness
- brought on by exertion
- relieved within five minutes by rest or glyceryl trinitrate.

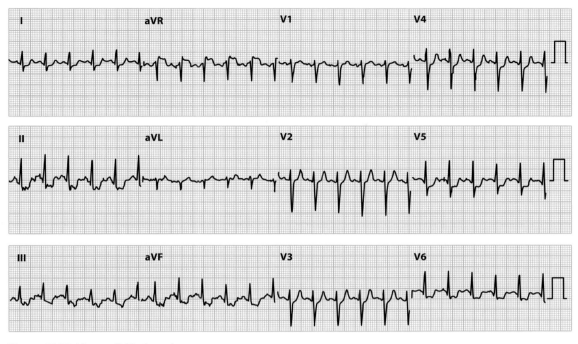

**Figure 15.15** Myocardial ischaemia.

Key point:    • There is inferolateral ST segment depression.

Patients with all three of these features are said to have 'typical angina', those with two features 'atypical angina', and those with one or no features 'non-anginal chest pain'.

The management of stable angina includes:

- modifying any risk factors (e.g. smoking, hypertension)
- aspirin, 75 mg once daily
- glyceryl trinitrate sublingually as required
- a statin
- consideration of an angiotensin-converting enzyme (ACE) inhibitor.

Add anti-anginal treatment as necessary to control symptoms:

- beta blocker
- calcium channel blocker
- long-acting oral or transdermal or buccal nitrate
- nicorandil
- ivabradine
- ranolazine.

If one or two anti-anginal drugs fail to control symptoms adequately, or if non-invasive investigations indicate that the patient is at high risk of an acute coronary syndrome, consider cardiac catheterization with a view to:

- percutaneous coronary intervention
- coronary artery bypass surgery.

Rapidly worsening chest pain, chest pain of recent onset or chest pain at rest in the context of ST segment depression indicates unstable angina or NSTEMI. This is a medical emergency, so urgent treatment is essential. Initial treatment options include:

- bedrest
- analgesia
- aspirin
- clopidogrel
- beta blockers
- intravenous or buccal nitrates
- antithrombotic therapy
- a glycoprotein IIb/IIIa inhibitor.

Patients with an acute coronary syndrome require risk stratification and, where appropriate, coronary angiography with a view to urgent intervention – discuss this with a cardiologist.

**ACT QUICKLY**

Acute coronary syndrome is a medical emergency. Prompt diagnosis and treatment are essential.

### Acute posterior myocardial infarction

Acute posterior myocardial infarction is discussed in Chapter 14. It is an ST segment *elevation* myocardial infarction (and the ST segment elevation can be seen if posterior chest leads, $V_7$–$V_9$, are recorded), but because the anterior chest leads $V_1$–$V_3$ have a reciprocal view of the infarction, these leads show ST segment *depression*, together with:

- dominant R waves
- upright, tall T waves.

An example is shown in Figure 14.4 (p. 149).

The management of acute posterior myocardial infarction is the same of that of other STEMIs, as outlined earlier in this chapter.

### 'Reciprocal' changes in ST segment elevation acute coronary syndrome

Just as acute posterior STEMI is associated with ST segment *depression* in the anterior chest leads ($V_1$–$V_3$), so any other STEMI can be associated with ST segment depression in leads that are 'distant' from the actual site of the myocardial event (Fig. 15.4, p. 163).

This phenomenon is seen in 30 per cent of anterior STEMIs and up to 80 per cent of inferior STEMIs, and the presence of reciprocal ST segment depression can be a useful pointer towards a diagnosis of STEMI where the implication of ST segment elevation is uncertain.

Although such ECG changes have traditionally been considered 'reciprocal' (i.e. a mirror image of electrical changes in the myocardium affected), there is some evidence that the ST segment depression is actually the result of ischaemia in a myocardial territory distant from the infarction site. The presence of 'reciprocal' ST segment depression in the context of STEMI is associated with more extensive coronary disease and carries a worse prognosis.

## Drugs

Digoxin has a characteristic effect on the ST segment, which is just one of its many effects on the whole ECG (Table 15.4). The ST segment depression seen with digoxin is described as a 'reverse tick' and is most obvious in leads with tall R waves (Fig. 15.16).

Always distinguish between digoxin *effects*, which may be apparent at therapeutic doses, and digoxin *toxicity*, which indicates overdosage. If digoxin toxicity is a possibility, ask about symptoms (anorexia, nausea, vomiting, abdominal pain and visual disturbance) and check the patient's digoxin and plasma potassium levels (arrhythmias are more likely if the patient is hypokalaemic).

Treat digoxin toxicity by stopping the drug and, where necessary, correcting potassium levels and treating arrhythmias. A digoxin-specific antibody may be used if the problem is life-threatening, but not without expert advice.

 **DRUG POINT**

A complete drug history is essential in any patient with an abnormal ECG.

**Table 15.4** Effects of digoxin on the ECG

At therapeutic levels:
- ST segment depression ('reverse tick')
- Reduction in T wave size
- Shortening of the QT interval

At toxic levels:
- T wave inversion
- Arrhythmias – almost any, but especially:
  - sinus bradycardia
  - paroxysmal atrial tachycardia with block
  - atrioventricular block
  - ventricular ectopics
  - ventricular bigeminy
  - ventricular tachycardia

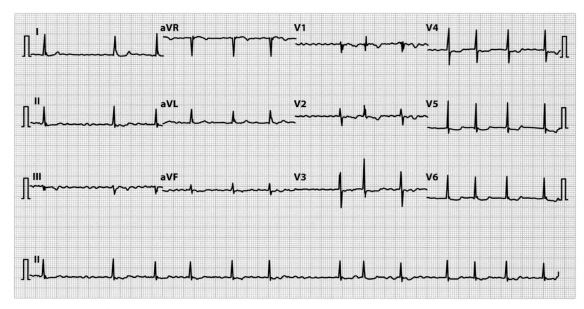

**Figure 15.16** Digoxin effect.

Key point:    • There is 'reverse tick' ST segment depression in the lateral leads.

## VENTRICULAR HYPERTROPHY WITH 'STRAIN'

The appearances of both left and right ventricular hypertrophy are discussed in Chapter 14. The 'strain' pattern is said to be present when, in addition to tall R waves and deep S waves, there is also:

● ST segment depression

● T wave inversion

in the leads that 'look at' the affected ventricle (Fig. 15.17).

The term 'strain' is rather misleading, because the underlying mechanism is unclear. If you see T wave inversion in the presence of other ECG evidence of ventricular hypertrophy, assess the patient carefully as described in Chapter 14, both for further evidence of ventricular hypertrophy and for an underlying cause.

### Are J waves present?

J waves, also known as Osborn waves, are typically seen in hypothermia (below 33°C). J waves have been reported to be present in around 80 per cent of ECGs in hypothermic patients, but they are also sometimes seen in patients with a normal body temperature and are therefore not completely specific for hypothermia.

The J wave is a small positive deflection at the junction between the QRS complex and the ST segment (Fig. 15.18) and is usually best seen in the inferior limb leads and the lateral chest leads.

Patients with hypothermia may also exhibit other ECG abnormalities, including AV block, atrial fibrillation, broadening of the QRS complexes, prolongation of the QT interval, ventricular arrhythmias and asystole.

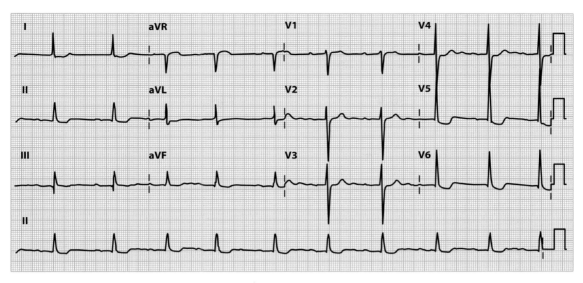

**Figure 15.17** Left ventricular hypertrophy with 'strain'.

Key point:    • There are tall R waves and deep S waves, with T wave inversion in leads $V_5$–$V_6$.

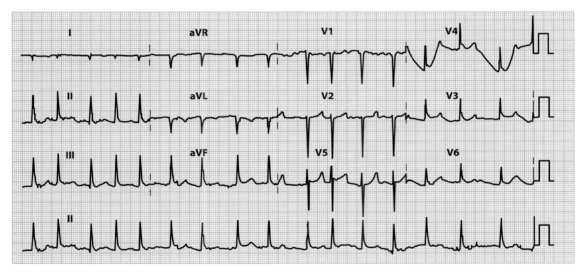

**Figure 15.18** J waves ('Osborn' waves) in hypothermia.

## SUMMARY

To assess the ST segment, ask the following questions:

*1. Are the ST segments elevated?*

If 'yes', consider:

- ST segment elevation myocardial infarction
- left ventricular aneurysm
- Prinzmetal's (vasospastic) angina

*(Continued)*

(*Continued*)
- pericarditis
- left bundle branch block
- Brugada syndrome
- high take-off.

*2. Are the ST segments depressed?*

If 'yes', consider:

- myocardial ischaemia
- acute posterior myocardial infarction
- 'reciprocal' changes in ST segment elevation myocardial infarction
- drugs (e.g. digoxin)
- ventricular hypertrophy with 'strain'.

*3. Are J waves present?*

If 'yes', consider:

- hypothermia.

## FURTHER READING

NICE guideline on chest pain of recent onset (2010). Downloadable from: http://guidance. nice.org.uk/CG95

NICE guideline on unstable angina and NSTEMI (2010). Downloadable from: http://guidance. nice.org.uk/CG94

Marinella MA. Electrocardiographic manifestations and differential diagnosis of acute pericarditis. *Am Fam Physician* 1998; 57: 699–704.

Rautaharju PM, Surawicz B, Gettes LS. AHA/ACCF/HRS recommendations for the standardization and interpretation of the electrocardiogram: Part IV: The ST segment, T and U waves, and the QT interval. *J Am Coll Cardiol* 2009; **53**: 982–991.

Sgarbossa EB, Pinski SL, Barbagelata A, *et al.* Electrocardiographic diagnosis of evolving acute myocardial infarction in the presence of left bundle-branch block. *N Engl J Med* 1996; **334**: 481–487.

# CHAPTER 16

# The T wave

After examining the ST segment, look carefully at the size and orientation of the T wave. The T wave corresponds to ventricular repolarization. The shape and orientation of normal T waves are shown in Figure 16.1.

It is normal for the T wave to be inverted in leads $V_1$ and aVR. In some cases, T wave inversion can also be normal in leads III and $V_2$, and sometimes even $V_3$, and these occurrences are discussed later in this chapter.

T waves can be abnormal in one of three ways, so the questions you need to ask about them are:

- Are the T waves too tall?
- Are the T waves too small?
- Are any of the T waves inverted?

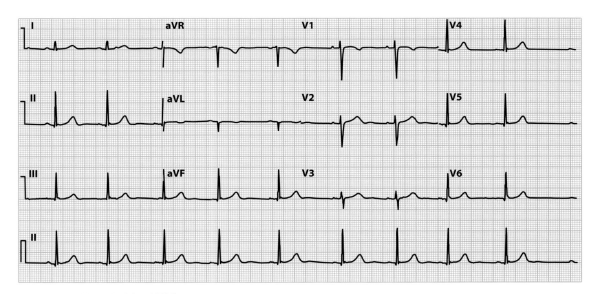

**Figure 16.1** Normal 12-lead ECG.

Key point:     • The shape and orientation of normal T waves varies from lead to lead.

## ARE THE T WAVES TOO TALL?

There is no clearly defined normal range for T wave height, although, as a general guide, a T wave should be no more than half the size of the preceding QRS complex. Your ability to recognize abnormally tall T waves will improve as you examine increasing numbers of ECGs and gain experience of the normal variations that occur.

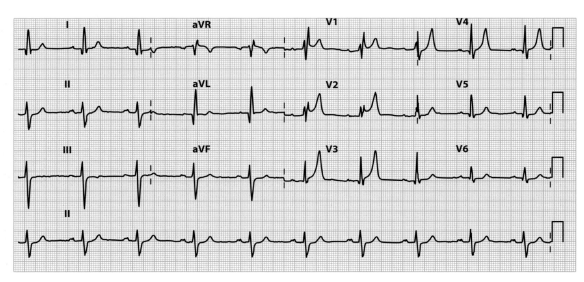

**Figure 16.2** Hyperkalaemia.

Key point:    • Tall 'tented' T waves are present in the anteroseptal chest leads.

If you suspect that the T waves are abnormally tall, consider whether your patient could have either of the following:

- hyperkalaemia
- acute coronary syndrome.

If either is a possibility, turn to the following pages for guidance on what to do next. Bear in mind, however, that tall T waves are often just a variant of normal, especially if you are judging just a single ECG. Your level of suspicion should be higher if you are comparing against earlier ECGs from the same patient and the height of the T waves has increased considerably.

## Hyperkalaemia

An elevated plasma potassium level can cause tall 'tented' T waves (Fig. 16.2).

Hyperkalaemia may also widen the T waves so that the entire ST segment is incorporated into the upstroke of the T wave. Hyperkalaemia may also cause:

- flattening and even loss of the P wave
- lengthening of the PR interval
- shortening of the QT interval
- widening of the QRS complex (Fig. 16.3), ultimately resembling a sine wave
- arrhythmias (ventricular fibrillation or asystole).

If the diagnosis is confirmed by a raised plasma potassium level, assess the patient for symptoms and signs of an underlying cause (e.g. renal failure). In particular, review their treatment chart for inappropriate potassium supplements and potassium-sparing diuretics.

**DRUG POINT**

A complete drug history is essential in any patient with an abnormal ECG.

16 The T wave

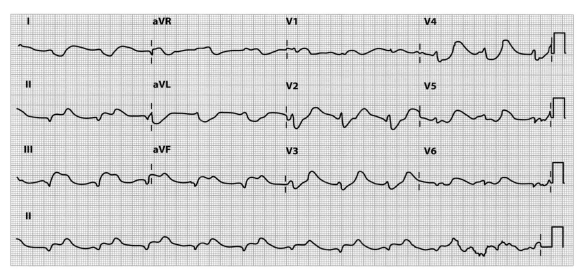

**Figure 16.3** Hyperkalaemia (severe).

Key point:    • P waves are absent and the QRS complexes are broad and 'bizarre' in appearance.

Because of the risk of fatal cardiac arrhythmias, hyperkalaemia needs *urgent* treatment if it is causing ECG abnormalities or the plasma potassium level is above 6.5 mmol/L.

**ACT QUICKLY**

Severe hyperkalaemia is a medical emergency. Prompt diagnosis and treatment are essential.

## Acute coronary syndrome

Tall 'hyperacute' T waves may be seen in the early stages of an acute coronary syndrome (Fig. 16.4). Increased T wave height may be a result of potassium released from damaged myocytes, leading to a localized hyperkalaemia.

Tall T waves are particularly characteristic of acute posterior myocardial infarction (p. 174). Infarction of the posterior wall of the left ventricle leads to reciprocal (i.e. 'mirror-image') changes when viewed from the perspective of the anterior chest leads. Thus, the usual myocardial infarction appearances of pathological Q waves, ST segment elevation and inverted T waves will appear as R waves, ST segment depression and upright, tall T waves when viewed from leads $V_1$–$V_3$.

The diagnosis and management of acute coronary syndrome are discussed in detail in Chapter 15.

**SEEK HELP**

Acute coronary syndromes require urgent treatment. Obtain the advice of a cardiologist without delay.

16 The T wave

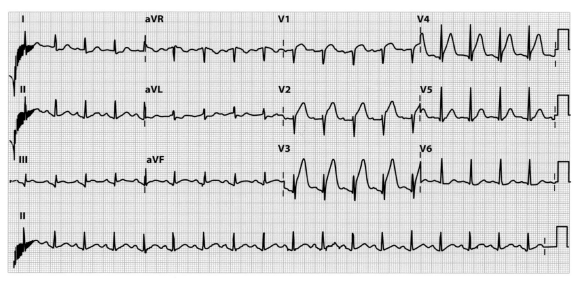

**Figure 16.4** Acute anterior myocardial infarction.

Key point:    • Tall 'hyperacute' T waves are present in the anteroseptal chest leads.

## ARE THE T WAVES TOO SMALL?

As with tall T waves, the judgement of whether T waves are abnormally small is subjective.

If you suspect that the T waves are abnormally small, consider whether your patient could have one of the following:

- hypokalaemia
- pericardial effusion
- hypothyroidism.

Advice about the diagnosis and treatment of each of these is given below.

### Hypokalaemia

Just as hyperkalaemia causes tall T waves, so hypokalaemia causes small T waves (Fig. 16.5).

Look carefully for other ECG changes that may accompany hypokalaemia:

- first-degree heart block
- depression of the ST segment
- prominent U waves.

If hypokalaemia is suspected, assess the patient for symptoms (e.g. muscle weakness, cramps) and review the treatment chart. Although many conditions can lead to hypokalaemia, the commonest cause is diuretics.

**DRUG POINT**

A complete drug history is essential in any patient with an abnormal ECG.

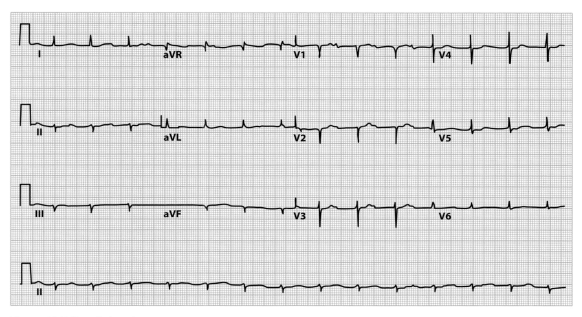

**Figure 16.5** Hypokalaemia.

Key point:    • There are small T waves and prominent U waves, plus first degree atrioventricular block and left axis deviation.

 **ACT QUICKLY**

Severe hypokalaemia is a medical emergency. Prompt diagnosis and treatment are essential.

## Pericardial effusion

If the whole ECG, and not just the T waves, is of a low voltage, think about the possibility of pericardial effusion. For a discussion of the investigation and treatment of pericardial effusion, see p. 151.

## Hypothyroidism

Hypothyroidism can cause small QRS complexes and small T waves, but the most characteristic finding is sinus bradycardia (p. 54). Perform a careful history and examination, and confirm the diagnosis with $T_3$, $T_4$ and thyroid-stimulating hormone levels.

## ARE ANY OF THE T WAVES INVERTED?

If T wave inversion is present, begin by asking:

• Could this be normal?

T wave inversion is considered normal in:

• leads aVR and $V_1$ (see Fig. 16.1)
• lead $V_2$ in younger people
• lead $V_3$ in black people.

T wave inversion in lead III can also be normal, and may be accompanied by a small Q wave – both of these findings can disappear if the ECG is repeated with the patient's breath held in deep inspiration.

T wave inversion in any other lead is generally considered abnormal, and if it is present, consider whether your patient has one of the following:

- myocardial ischaemia
- myocardial infarction
- ventricular hypertrophy with 'strain'
- digoxin effect.

You will find advice about the recognition and management of each of these conditions below.

There are also several conditions in which T wave inversion occurs in combination with other ECG abnormalities. If the ECG has been normal up to this point of the assessment, it is unlikely that any of the following are to blame for the T wave inversion. Nonetheless, if you still have not found a cause after going through the list above, consider:

- repolarization abnormalities following a paroxysmal tachycardia
- bundle branch block (Chapters 9 and 14)
- pericarditis (Chapter 15)
- ventricular pacing (Chapter 20).

Finally, there are four conditions in which T wave inversion can occur but the ECG is not diagnostic:

- hyperventilation
- mitral valve prolapse
- pulmonary embolism
- subarachnoid haemorrhage.

If your patient has one of these conditions, you do not need to look for another cause of T wave inversion unless there are other reasons to suspect one.

## Myocardial ischaemia

ST segment depression is the commonest manifestation of myocardial ischaemia (Chapter 15), but T wave inversion may also occur in the leads that 'look at' the affected areas (Fig. 16.6). Because ischaemia is reversible, these ECG abnormalities will only be observed during an ischaemic episode.

Patients whose T waves are inverted to begin with (e.g. following a myocardial infarction) may develop temporarily upright T waves during ischaemic episodes. This is referred to as T wave 'pseudonormalization'.

The management of myocardial ischaemia is described in detail on page 172.

### WELLENS' SIGN

Wellens' sign (also known as Wellens' syndrome or 'Wellens' warning') can be seen during an episode of unstable angina in patients with a severe, often critical, proximal stenosis of the left anterior descending coronary artery. It is characterized by symmetrical, deep (>2 mm) T wave inversion in the anterior chest leads (Fig. 16.7). Patients with Wellens' sign should be referred urgently for coronary angiography as there is a significant risk of going on to sustain an anterior myocardial infarction.

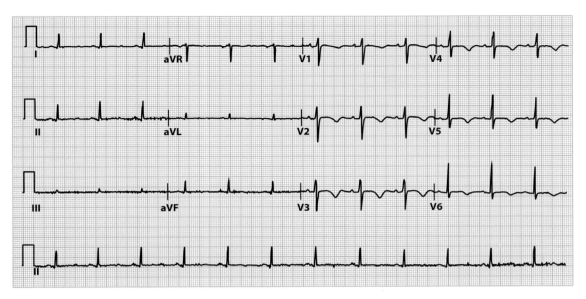

**Figure 16.6** Myocardial ischaemia.

Key points:
- Abnormal T wave inversion (leads $V_2$–$V_6$) during an episode of myocardial ischaemia.
- There is also, incidentally, prolongation of the QT interval.

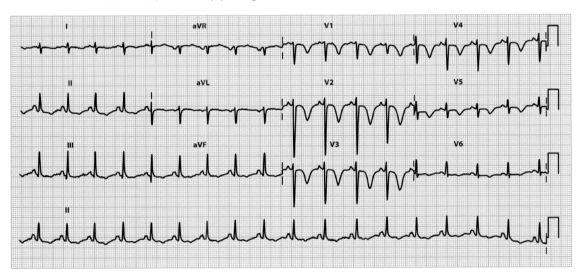

**Figure 16.7** Wellens' sign.

Key points:
- Deep T wave inversion in the anterior chest leads in a patient presenting with unstable angina.
- Coronary angiography revealed a critical proximal stenosis in the left anterior descending coronary artery.

## Myocardial infarction

T wave inversion can occur not only as a temporary change in myocardial ischaemia but also as a more prolonged (and sometimes permanent) change in myocardial infarction. In Chapter 15, we mentioned that myocardial infarctions are often divided into:

- ST segment elevation myocardial infarction (STEMI)
- non-ST segment elevation myocardial infarction (NSTEMI).

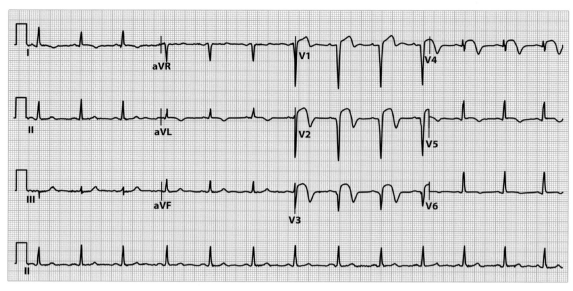

**Figure 16.8** Evolving ST segment elevation myocardial infarction.

Key points:
* As the ST segment elevation returns to baseline, T wave inversion develops.
* Note also the development of Q waves in the anterior leads.

T wave inversion can occur in either type of infarct. In STEMI, the T wave inversion accompanies the return of the elevated ST segment to baseline (Fig. 16.8). T wave inversion may be permanent, or the T wave may return to normal. NSTEMI can also cause T wave inversion, although it can also manifest as ST segment depression alone.

If you see abnormal T wave inversion on an ECG, question the patient about any history of chest pain and previous angina or myocardial infarctions and assess their risk factors for cardiovascular disease (see Table 15.1, p. 160).

The management of acute coronary syndrome is detailed in Chapter 15.

 **ACT QUICKLY**

Acute coronary syndrome is a medical emergency. Prompt diagnosis and treatment are essential.

## Ventricular hypertrophy with 'strain'

In addition to tall R waves and deep S waves, ventricular hypertrophy can also cause ST segment depression and T wave inversion. This is commonly referred to as a 'strain' pattern (p. 176).

If present, the 'strain' pattern is seen in the leads that 'look at' the hypertrophied ventricle. With left ventricular hypertrophy the abnormalities will be seen in leads I, aVL and $V_4$–$V_6$ (Fig. 16.9). Right ventricular hypertrophy causes changes in leads $V_1$–$V_3$.

The term 'strain' is rather misleading because the underlying mechanism is unclear. Although some conditions, such as massive pulmonary embolism, can certainly place a ventricle under an increased workload and are associated with the 'strain' pattern, it is also seen in cases of ventricular hypertrophy where there is no apparent stress on the ventricle.

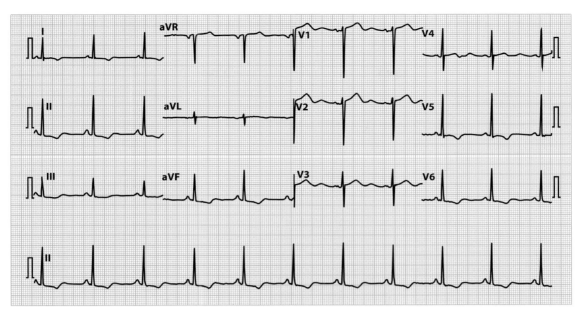

**Figure 16.9** Left ventricular hypertrophy with 'strain'.

Key point:    • As well as large QRS complexes, T wave inversion is present in the lateral leads.

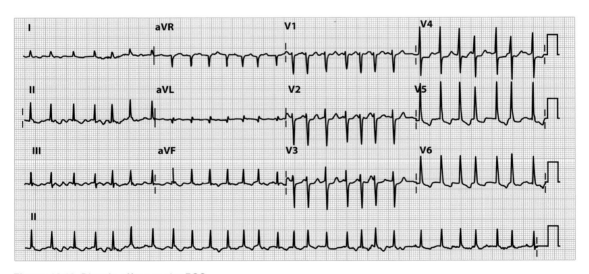

**Figure 16.10** Digoxin effect on the ECG.

Key point:    • There is reverse tick ST segment depression and T wave inversion in leads $V_5$–$V_6$. Patient on digoxin for atrial fibrillation with a very fast ventricular rate (168/min).

If you see T wave inversion in the presence of other ECG evidence of ventricular hypertrophy, assess the patient carefully as described in Chapter 14.

## Digoxin effect

As well as causing 'reverse tick' ST segment depression (Fig. 15.16), digoxin can also cause T wave inversion (Fig. 16.10).

Always distinguish between digoxin effects, which may be apparent at therapeutic doses, and digoxin toxicity, which indicates overdosage. If digoxin toxicity is a possibility, ask about symptoms (anorexia, nausea, vomiting, abdominal pain and visual disturbance) and check the patient's digoxin and plasma potassium levels (arrhythmias are more likely if the patient is hypokalaemic).

**DRUG POINT**

A complete drug history is essential in any patient with an abnormal ECG.

## SUMMARY

To assess the T wave, ask the following questions:

*1. Are the T waves too tall?*

If 'yes', consider:

- hyperkalaemia
- acute coronary syndrome.

*2. Are the T waves too small?*

If 'yes', consider:

- hypokalaemia
- pericardial effusion
- hypothyroidism.

*3. Are any of the T waves inverted?*

If 'yes', consider:

- normal (leads aVR and $V_1$)
- normal variant (leads $V_2$, $V_3$ and III)
- myocardial ischaemia
- myocardial infarction
- ventricular hypertrophy with 'strain'
- digoxin effect.

Also bear in mind:

- repolarization abnormalities following a paroxysmal tachycardia
- bundle branch block (Chapters 9 and 14)
- pericarditis (Chapter 15)
- ventricular pacing (Chapter 20)
- hyperventilation
- mitral valve prolapse
- pulmonary embolism
- subarachnoid haemorrhage.

16 The T wave

## FURTHER READING

Mead NE, O'Keefe KP. Wellens' syndrome: an ominous EKG pattern. *J Emerg Trauma Shock* 2009; **2**: 206–208.

Montague BT, Ouellette JR, Buller GK. Retrospective review of the frequency of ECG changes in hyperkalemia. *Clin J Am Soc Nephrol* 2008; **3**: 324–330.

Rautaharju PM, Surawicz B, Gettes LS. AHA/ACCF/HRS recommendations for the standardization and interpretation of the electrocardiogram: Part IV: The ST segment, T and U waves, and the QT interval. *J Am Coll Cardiol* 2009; **53**: 982–991.

Wagner GS, Macfarlane P, Wellens H, *et al.* AHA/ACCF/HRS recommendations for the standardization and interpretation of the electrocardiogram: Part VI: Acute ischaemia/infarction. *J Am Coll Cardiol* 2009; **53**: 1003–1011.

After examining the T waves, measure the QT interval. This is the time from the *start* of the QRS complex to the *end* of the T wave (Fig. 17.1), and it represents the total duration of electrical activity (depolarization and repolarization) in the ventricles.

The QT interval varies slightly between leads, and so in general the lead with the **longest** QT interval is taken for the measurement. Usually, this will be lead $V_2$ or $V_3$. When determining the duration of the QT interval, it is important to measure it to the end of the T wave and not the U wave (if one is present – see Chapter 18). It is easy to mistake a U wave for a T wave and thus overestimate the QT interval. If U waves are present and you are struggling to differentiate between the end of the T wave and the U wave, you may find it easier to make the measurement in lead aVR or aVL, in which the U waves are usually least prominent.

As with any interval in the ECG, there are only two possible abnormalities of the QT interval:

- the QT interval can be too long
- the QT interval can be too short.

Unfortunately, deciding whether or not the QT interval is normal is not entirely straightforward, because the duration varies according to the patient's heart rate: the faster the heart rate, the shorter the QT interval. To allow for this, you must calculate the corrected QT interval ($QT_c$). The most commonly used formula for doing so is **Bazett's formula** (see box):

$$QT_c = \frac{QT}{\sqrt{RR}}$$

where $QT_c$ is the corrected QT interval, QT is the measured QT interval and RR is the measured RR interval (all measurements in seconds).

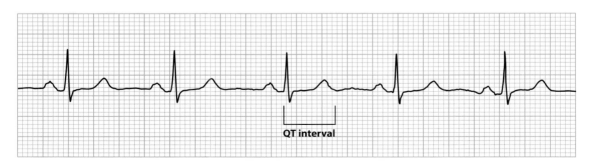

**Figure 17.1** The QT interval.

Key point:   • The QT interval is 380 msec in this patient.

Bazett's formula has limitations, and tends to overcorrect or undercorrect the QT interval at extremes of heart rate. Other formulae are also used, and so-called linear formulae tend to be more uniform over a wide range of heart rates.

The normal upper limit of the $QT_c$ interval is 450 msec in men and 460 msec in women. The lower limit of the $QT_c$ interval is 390 msec (in both sexes). However, it is worth noting that there is not an absolutely clear cut-off between 'normal' and 'abnormal', and results just on either side of these values could be regarded as borderline.

When you assess the QT interval, therefore, ask yourself the following two questions:

- Is the $QT_c$ interval long?
- Is the $QT_c$ interval short?

If the answer to either question is 'yes', turn to the relevant section of this chapter to find out what to do next. If 'no', you can move on to the next chapter.

### WHY CORRECT THE QT INTERVAL?

Correction of the QT interval is necessary because the normal QT interval varies with heart rate: the faster the heart rate, the shorter the normal QT interval. Although graphs and tables of normal QT intervals at different heart rates are available, it is inconvenient to have to look up the normal range every time you want to check someone's QT interval.

An alternative way to assess a QT interval is to correct it to what it would be if the patient's heart rate was 60 beats/min. By doing this, all you will then need to remember is one normal range for the QT interval.

You will need a pocket calculator to calculate the corrected QT interval ('$QT_c$ interval'). Divide the patient's measured QT interval (measured in seconds) by the square root of their RR interval (also measured in seconds). This is Bazett's formula:

$$QT_c = \frac{QT}{\sqrt{RR}}$$

The RR interval is the time between consecutive R waves, and can be either measured directly from the ECG or calculated by dividing 60 by the patient's heart rate. For example, at a heart rate of 80 beats/min the RR interval is 0.75 s.

Many of the more sophisticated ECG machines automatically print out a value for the $QT_c$ interval on the ECG. However, always check for yourself values that are automatically measured in this way, as errors do occur.

The normal upper limit for the QT interval at a heart rate of 60 beats/min, and thus for the $QT_c$ interval, is 0.45 s (450 msec) in men and 0.46 s (460 msec) in women.

## IS THE $QT_c$ INTERVAL LONG?

If the $QT_c$ interval is >450 msec in men and >460 msec in women, then the patient's corrected QT interval is prolonged (Fig. 17.2). The causes you need to consider are:

- hypocalcaemia
- drug effects

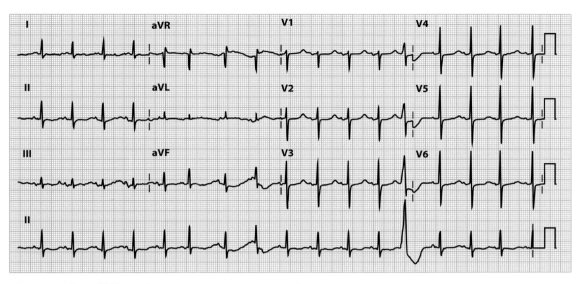

**Figure 17.2** Long QT interval.

Key points:
- The measured QT interval is 440 msec.
- The heart rate is 102 beats/min, $QT_c$ interval is 574 msec.

- acute myocarditis
- long QT syndrome.

If any of these is a possibility, consult the following pages to find out what to do next.

In addition, there are also several conditions in which QT interval prolongation is recognized, but in which this abnormality is an interesting feature rather than a useful diagnostic pointer. Such conditions include:

- acute myocardial infarction
- cerebral injury
- hypertrophic cardiomyopathy
- hypothermia.

You simply need to be aware that QT interval prolongation is recognized in these conditions, so that you do not need to look for another cause unless clinically suspected.

## Hypocalcaemia

Hypocalcaemia is a well-recognized cause of QT interval prolongation. The clinical features (peripheral and circumoral paraesthesiae, tetany, fits and psychiatric disturbance) are characteristic. Look for Trousseau's sign (carpal spasm when the brachial artery is occluded with a blood-pressure cuff), Chvostek's sign (twitching of facial muscles when tapping over the facial nerve) and papilloedema. Confirm the diagnosis by checking a plasma calcium level on an uncuffed blood sample, not forgetting to check a simultaneous albumin level so that any necessary correction can be made.

Once a diagnosis of hypocalcaemia has been made, always look for the underlying cause (Table 17.1).

Table 17.1 Causes of hypocalcaemia

- Hypoparathyroidism
  - following thyroid surgery
  - autoimmune
  - congenital (DiGeorge's syndrome)
- Pseudohypoparathyroidism
- Chronic renal failure
- Vitamin D deficiency/resistance
- Drugs (e.g. calcitonin)
- Acute pancreatitis

The treatment of hypocalcaemia depends on the severity of symptoms. Treat severe hypocalcaemia with intravenous calcium (given as 10 mL calcium gluconate 10 per cent). Treat those who have milder symptoms with oral calcium supplements and, if necessary, oral vitamin D derivatives. Carefully monitor plasma calcium levels to avoid over-treatment and consequent hypercalcaemia.

## Drug effects

Several anti-arrhythmic drugs cause prolongation of the QT interval by slowing myocardial conduction, and thus repolarization. Examples are quinidine, procainamide and flecainide. QT interval prolongation is also seen with terfenadine and tricyclic antidepressants.

Drug-induced QT interval prolongation is associated with torsades de pointes (Chapter 8), which can lead to ventricular fibrillation and sudden cardiac death. The problem therefore requires immediate attention, and referral to a cardiologist for review of anti-arrhythmic drug treatment is recommended.

**DRUG POINT**

A complete drug history is essential in any patient with an abnormal ECG.

## Acute myocarditis

QT interval prolongation can occur with any cause of acute myocarditis, although it is usually associated with rheumatic carditis.

Presenting features often include a fever, chest discomfort, palpitations and symptoms of heart failure (dyspnoea and fatigue). Examination may reveal quiet heart sounds, a friction rub, tachycardia, a fourth heart sound and gallop rhythm. There may also be features specific to the underlying cause (Table 17.2).

Other ECG changes may be present, including:

- ST segment changes
- T wave inversion
- heart block (of any degree of severity)
- arrhythmias.

A chest X-ray may show cardiomegaly. A cardiac biopsy reveals acute inflammatory changes, and the levels of cardiac enzymes will be raised. Rarely, viral serology may establish the aetiology.

**Table 17.2** Causes of myocarditis

- Infectious
  - viral (e.g. coxsackie, influenza)
  - bacterial (e.g. acute rheumatic fever, diphtheria)
  - protozoal (e.g. Chagas' disease, toxoplasmosis)
  - rickettsial
- Drug induced (e.g. chloroquine)
- Toxic agents (e.g. lead)
- Peripartum

The treatment of acute myocarditis is supportive. Bedrest is recommended. Treat heart failure, arrhythmias and heart block as necessary. Antibiotics are indicated where a responsive organism is suspected. Although many patients will go on to make a good recovery, some are left with heart failure.

**SEEK HELP**

Acute myocarditis requires specialist assessment. Obtain the advice of a cardiologist without delay.

## Long QT syndrome

Many hereditary syndromes are now recognized in which an abnormality of the sodium or potassium ion channels causes a susceptibility to ventricular arrhythmias and sudden cardiac death. These syndromes include **long QT syndrome** (LQTS), in which genetic abnormalities of the potassium or sodium channels lead to prolonged ventricular repolarization and hence prolongation of the QT interval.

Several genetic abnormalities have now been identified, the three most common being termed LQT1 and LQT2 (potassium channel abnormalities) and LQT3 (sodium channel abnormality). The classification of LQTS includes the hereditary syndromes:

- Romano–Ward syndrome
- Jervell and Lange-Nielsen syndrome.

The autosomal dominant Romano–Ward syndrome consists of recurrent syncopal attacks and sudden death secondary to ventricular tachycardia, torsades de pointes and ventricular fibrillation. The arrhythmias are often triggered by exercise or stress.

The autosomal recessive Jervell and Lange-Nielsen syndrome is much rarer and carries the same risk of ventricular arrhythmias. Unlike the Romano–Ward syndrome, it is also associated with congenital high-tone deafness.

Patients with long QT syndrome need careful risk assessment and will usually require anti-arrhythmic medication (commonly beta-blockers). Those at high risk of ventricular arrhythmias will usually need an implantable cardioverter defibrillator.

**SEEK HELP**

Long QT syndrome is potentially life-threatening. Obtain the advice of a cardiologist without delay.

## IS THE QT$_C$ INTERVAL SHORT?

If the QT$_c$ is <390 msec, the patient's corrected QT interval is shorter than normal and you should check for the following:

- congenital short QT syndromes
- hypercalcaemia
- hyperkalaemia
- digoxin effect.

If any of these is a possibility, read below to find out what to do next.

Shortening of the QT$_c$ interval is also recognized in hyperthermia. Having established the diagnosis of hyperthermia clinically, you will not need to look for another cause for a shortened QT$_c$ interval unless there is a good reason to do so.

### Congenital short QT syndromes

Although congenital long QT syndromes are well recognized, it is only in the past few years that congenital short QT syndromes have been clearly described. The congenital short QT syndromes appear to follow an autosomal dominant pattern of inheritance and mutations affecting the genes *KCNH2*, *KCNQ1* and *KCNJ2* (which are linked to potassium channels) and *CACNA1C* and *CACNB2B* (which are linked to calcium channels) have so far been identified.

Most patients have inducible ventricular fibrillation on electrophysiological testing and a family history of sudden cardiac death or atrial fibrillation. The QT$_c$ interval is usually very short indeed, and the diagnosis should be certainly considered on finding a QT$_c$ interval below 330 msec.

Implantation of a cardioverter defibrillator forms the cornerstone of treatment, although this can be challenging in view of the very young age at which the condition is diagnosed in some individuals. Drug treatment (e.g. quinidine) to lengthen the QT interval may be possible, depending upon the subtype of short QT syndrome. The management of this condition is complex and requires the input of a cardiologist with a special interest in arrhythmias.

**SEEK HELP**

Congenital short QT syndromes are potentially life threatening. Obtain the advice of a cardiologist without delay.

### Hypercalcaemia

The shortened QT interval in hypercalcaemia results from abnormally rapid ventricular repolarization (Fig. 17.3).

Symptoms of hypercalcaemia include anorexia, weight loss, nausea, vomiting, abdominal pain, constipation, polydipsia, polyuria, weakness and depression.

A prominent U wave may also be seen in hypercalcaemia. Confirm the diagnosis with a plasma calcium level (correcting the result for the patient's current albumin level). The underlying causes that you need to consider are listed in Table 17.3.

The treatment of hypercalcaemia depends, in the long term, on the underlying cause. Immediate management depends on the symptoms and plasma calcium level. There is a risk of cardiac arrest with severe hypercalcaemia, so prompt recognition and treatment are essential.

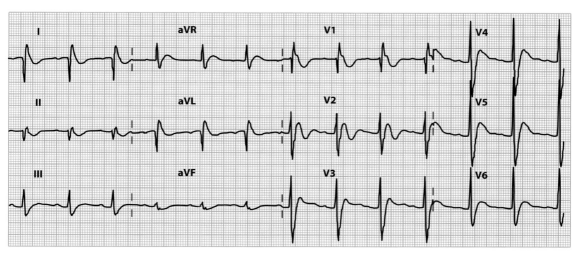

**Figure 17.3** Short QT interval in hypercalcaemia.

Key points:
- The measured QT interval is 300 msec.
- The heart rate is 73 beats/min, $QT_c$ interval is 331 msec.

**Table 17.3** Causes of hypercalcaemia

- Hyperparathyroidism
  - primary
  - tertiary
- Malignancy (including myeloma)
- Drugs
  - thiazide diuretics
  - excessive vitamin D intake
- Sarcoidosis
- Thyrotoxicosis
- Milk–Alkali Syndrome

Severe symptoms (e.g. vomiting, drowsiness) or a plasma calcium level greater than 3.5 mmol/L warrant urgent treatment as follows:

- intravenous 0.9 per cent saline (e.g. 3–4 L/24 h)
- intravenous furosemide (20–40 mg every 6–12 h *after rehydration*)
- bisphosphonates (e.g. disodium pamidronate – single infusion of 30 mg over 2 h)
- discontinuation of thiazides/vitamin D compounds
- monitoring of urea and electrolytes and calcium levels every 12 h.

 **ACT QUICKLY**

Severe hypercalcaemia is a medical emergency. Prompt diagnosis and treatment are essential.

## Hyperkalaemia

Hyperkalaemia can cause a number of abnormalities on the ECG, of which shortening of the QT interval is one. Turn to page 180 to read more about the ECG changes seen in hyperkalaemia.

17 The QT interval

## Digoxin effect

Shortening of the QT interval is one of several effects that treatment with digoxin has on the ECG (see Table 15.4, p. 175). It is important to note that digoxin *effects* are normal, and do not imply that the patient has digoxin *toxicity*. The effects of digoxin on the ECG are covered in more detail in Chapter 15.

**DRUG POINT**

A complete drug history is essential in any patient with an abnormal ECG.

## SUMMARY

To assess the QT interval, ask the following questions:

*1. Is the $QT_c$ interval long?*

If 'yes', consider:

- hypocalcaemia
- drug effects
- acute myocarditis
- long QT syndrome.

Also bear in mind:

- acute myocardial infarction
- cerebral injury
- hypertrophic cardiomyopathy
- hypothermia.

*2. Is the $QT_c$ interval short?*

If 'yes', consider:

- hereditary short QT syndromes
- hypercalcaemia
- hyperkalaemia
- digoxin effect.

Also bear in mind:

- hyperthermia.

## FURTHER READING

Giustetto C, Di Monte F, Wolpert C, *et al*. Short QT syndrome: clinical findings and diagnostic-therapeutic implications. *Eur Heart J* 2006; **27**: 2440–2447.

Goldenberg I, Moss AJ. Long QT syndrome. *J Am Coll Cardiol* 2008; **51**: 2291–2300.

Rautaharju PM, Surawicz B, Gettes LS. AHA/ACCF/HRS recommendations for the standardization and interpretation of the electrocardiogram: Part IV: The ST segment, T and U waves, and the QT interval. *J Am Coll Cardiol* 2009; **53**: 982–991.

# CHAPTER 18

# The U wave

The U wave follows the T wave (Fig. 18.1) and is most clearly visible in the anterior chest leads $V_2$–$V_3$ (Fig. 18.2). U waves are more commonly seen when patients are bradycardic: U waves are commonly visible at heart rates <65 beats/min, but are seldom seen at heart rates >95 beats/min.

Over a century ago, Einthoven said that 'the significance of [the U wave] and the reason for its inconstancy are for the present not known with surety'. The same is still true today – there continues to be considerable debate about the origin of the U wave, although many theories exist.

It has been suggested that the U wave represents repolarization of the interventricular septum, or of the Purkinje fibres, or of the papillary muscles, or of myocytes in the mid-myocardium (so-called 'M cells'). It has also been suggested that the U wave is caused by after-potentials following the cardiac action potential, or that it is really just a continuation of the T wave, and that T and U waves should both be considered together as part of the overall process of ventricular repolarization.

Normally, U waves are small and point in the same direction as the preceding T wave. When you assess the U wave, ask the following questions:

- Do the U waves appear too prominent?
- Are any of the U waves inverted?

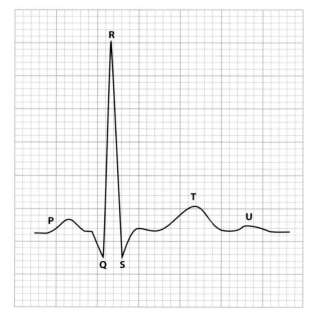

**Figure 18.1** The U wave.

| Key point: | • The U wave follows the T wave. |
| --- | --- |

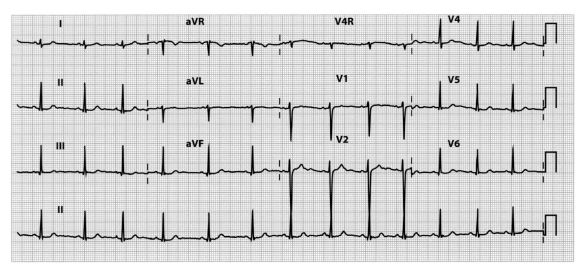

**Figure 18.2** Prominent U waves.

Key point:    • U waves are best seen in lead V₂ (note atypical lead layout on the ECG).

## DO THE U WAVES APPEAR TOO PROMINENT?

This is not a straightforward question to answer, because there is no normal range that you can apply to the height of a U wave (although they are generally <25% of the height of the preceding T wave). Suspecting the U waves are too prominent depends to a degree on subjective judgement rather than objective measurement, and there is no substitute for reporting large numbers of ECGs to gain experience of the range of normality of the U wave (and, for that matter, all other aspects of the ECG). Remember that U waves tend to be more prominent when patients are bradycardic, so be aware that a prominent U wave may simply reflect a patient's low heart rate.

It follows on from all this that you should not attach too much weight to U wave prominence. Simply regard it as a clue that it may be due to one of the following:

● hypokalaemia
● drugs.

If either of these is a possibility, turn to the appropriate section of this chapter to find out what to do next.

### Hypokalaemia

Prominent U waves can be just one of a number of ECG abnormalities seen in the hypokalaemic patient (Fig. 18.2). Other associated ECG changes include:

● first-degree atrioventricular block (Chapter 9)
● depression of the ST segment (Chapter 15)
● small T waves (Chapter 16).

The investigation and treatment of hypokalaemia are discussed in detail on page 182.

**BE ALERT!**

In severe hypokalaemia (serum potassium <2.7 mmol/L), the size of the U wave may exceed that of the T wave. Therefore, if you see U waves that are larger than T waves on an ECG, check the patient's serum potassium level urgently. Prompt diagnosis and treatment are essential.

## Drugs

A number of anti-arrhythmic drugs can make the U wave more prominent:

- Class Ia anti-arrhythmics (e.g. quinidine, procainamide)
- Class III anti-arrhythmics (e.g. amiodarone, sotalol)
- digoxin.

If you see prominent U waves, check the patient's drug history to see if their medication may be the reason.

## ARE ANY OF THE U WAVES INVERTED?

U waves normally point in the same direction as the preceding T wave, and so U wave inversion is abnormal if the accompanying T wave is upright. Over 90% of patients with U wave inversion have some form of cardiovascular pathology, most commonly:

- ischaemic heart disease
- hypertension
- valvular regurgitation
- dilated cardiomyopathy.

The finding of U wave inversion should therefore prompt a review of the patient's history and examination (and further investigation where appropriate) for evidence of these cardiovascular conditions.

---

SUMMARY

To assess the U wave, ask the following questions:

*1. Do the U waves appear too prominent?*

If 'yes', consider:

- hypokalaemia
- drugs.

*2. Are any of the U waves inverted?*

If 'yes', consider:

- ischaemic heart disease
- hypertension
- valvular regurgitation
- dilated cardiomyopathy.

---

## FURTHER READING

Conrath CE, Opthof T. The patient U wave. *Cardiovasc Res* 2005; **67**: 184–186.

Correale E, Battista R, Ricciardiello V, *et al*. The negative U wave: A pathogenetic enigma but a useful, often overlooked bedside diagnostic and prognostic clue in ischemic heart disease. *Clin Cardiol* 2004; **27**: 674–677.

di Bernardo D, Murray A. Origin on the electrocardiogram of U-waves and abnormal U-wave inversion. *Cardiovasc Res* 2002; **53**: 202–208.

Rautaharju PM, Surawicz B, Gettes LS. AHA/ACCF/HRS recommendations for the standardization and interpretation of the electrocardiogram: Part IV: The ST segment, T and U waves, and the QT interval. *J Am Coll Cardiol* 2009; **53**: 982–991.

Ritsema van Eck HJ, Kors JA, van Herpen G. The U wave in the electrocardiogram: a solution for a 100-year-old riddle. *Cardiovasc Res* 2005; **67**: 256–262.

If you encounter ECG abnormalities that appear atypical or that do not fit with the patient's clinical condition, always consider the possibility that they may be artefacts caused by:

- electrode misplacement
- external electrical interference
- incorrect calibration
- incorrect paper speed
- patient movement.

Examples of each of these are discussed on the following pages.

**REMEMBER**

- Never give undue weight to a single investigation, particularly if the result does not fit with your clinical findings.
- Do not hesitate to repeat an ECG if you suspect that the abnormalities could be artefacts.

## ELECTRODE MISPLACEMENT

The correct position of each recording electrode is given in Chapter 3. It can be quite easy to swap two electrodes inadvertently; this is particularly common with the limb electrodes.

Figure 19.1 shows an ECG recorded with the two arm electrodes swapped over. The abnormalities can be quite subtle, but you should always think of electrode misplacement if you see unexpected wave inversions.

## EXTERNAL ELECTRICAL INTERFERENCE

External electrical interference (e.g. from electrical appliances) seldom causes difficulties when recording ECGs in hospital. However, for general practitioners who sometimes record ECGs in patients' homes, 50 Hz electrical interference from domestic appliances has been reported as a major cause of ECG artefact, and this can make the ECG difficult or even impossible to interpret correctly.

Always bear this in mind when interpreting an ECG recorded in a patient's home. Unless the source of the interference can be identified and removed, there is little that can be done apart from repeating the recording with the patient in a new location.

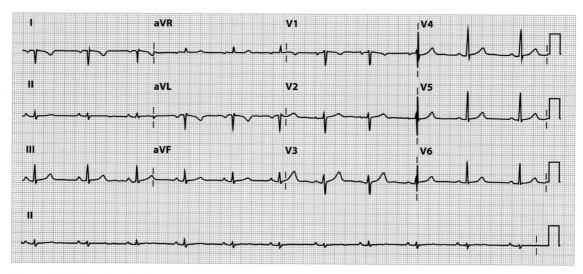

**Figure 19.1** Electrode misplacement.

Key points:
- The left and right arm electrodes have been swapped over.
- The QRS complexes in leads I and aVL are negative, and the P waves and T waves are inverted in leads I and aVL.
- There is extreme right axis deviation (+152°), and a positive QRS complex in lead aVR. Note that similar appearances may be seen in the limb leads in dextrocardia, but dextrocardia would also show abnormal chest leads.

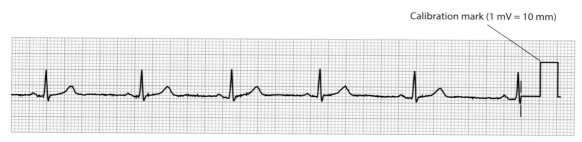

Calibration mark (1 mV = 10 mm)

**Figure 19.2** Correct calibration.

Key point:
- Note the 10 mm calibration mark (1 mV = 10 mm).

## INCORRECT CALIBRATION

The standard ECG is recorded so that a voltage of 1 mV makes the recording needle move 10 mm (1 cm). Every ECG must include a calibration mark (Fig. 19.2) so that the gain setting can be checked. If you see waves that appear too big or too small, always double-check the size of the calibration mark (Fig. 19.3).

Sometimes it is necessary to alter the gain setting, particularly if the QRS complexes are so big at the standard setting that they will not fit clearly on the paper. If it is necessary to change to a non-standard calibration, it is good practice to highlight this clearly by writing a note on the ECG.

19 Artefacts on the ECG

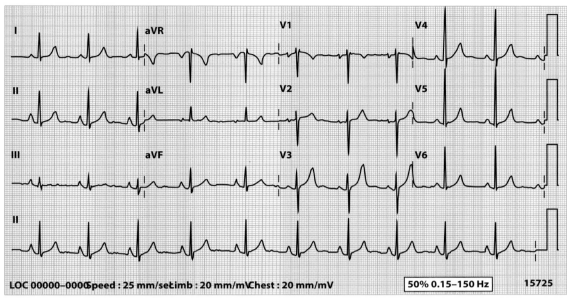

**Figure 19.3** Incorrect calibration.

Key point:   • The voltage calibration has been set at 20 mm/mV (double the standard setting of 10 mm/mV) and so all the waves/complexes appear twice their 'usual' size.

## INCORRECT PAPER SPEED

In the UK and USA, the standard ECG recording speed is 25 mm/s, so that 1 small (1 mm) square equals 0.04 s. If the paper is run at double the speed (50 mm/s, which is standard in some parts of Europe), the waves will double in width (Fig. 19.4). Always label every ECG you record with the paper speed used and, if you use a non-standard setting, it is good practice to highlight this clearly at the top of the ECG.

## PATIENT MOVEMENT

The ECG records the electrical activity of the heart, but this is not the only source of electrical activity in the body. Skeletal muscle activity is also picked up on the ECG (Fig. 19.5), and it is important for patients to lie still and relaxed while an ECG is being recorded. Unfortunately, this is not always possible, particularly if the patient:

● is uncooperative or agitated

● is in respiratory distress

● has a movement disorder.

Skeletal muscle activity is unavoidable during exercise testing. The use of signal-averaged ECGs, which 'average out' random electrical artefacts by combining a number of PQRST complexes, can help (Fig. 19.6). However, signal-averaged recordings can also be misleading by introducing artefactual changes of their own, and such recordings should always be interpreted with discretion.

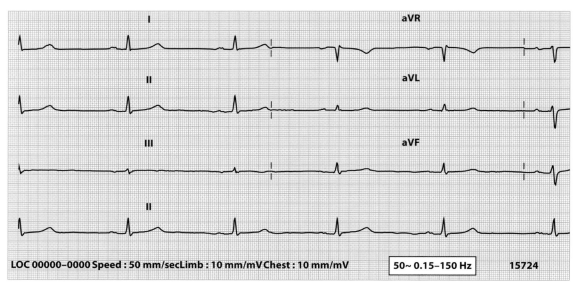

**Figure 19.4** Paper speed and wave width.

Key point:    • Waves are wider at higher paper speeds, in this case 50 mm/s.

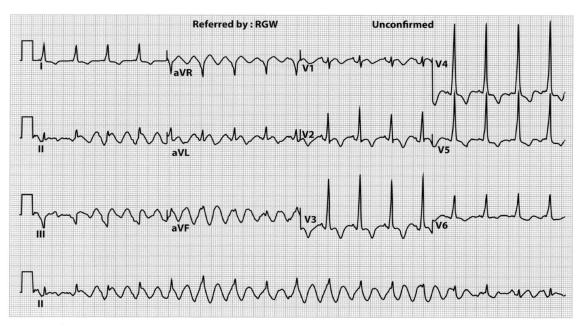

**Figure 19.5** Movement artefact.

Key points:    • Rhythmic abnormal movement of the limbs in Parkinson's disease is seen as a regular artefact on the ECG.
   • On careful inspection, the QRS complexes can still be seen within this artefact (best appreciated in the rhythm strip, lead II).

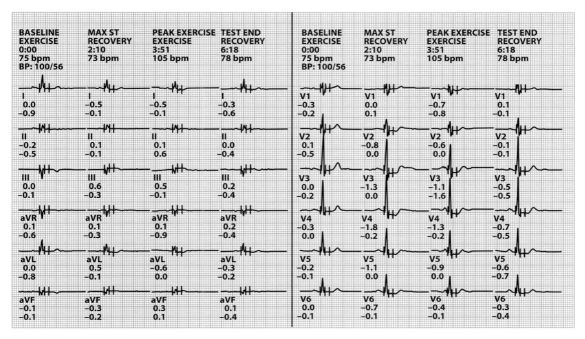

**Figure 19.6** Signal-averaged ECG.

Key points:
- Electrical artefacts are reduced by signal averaging.
- These signal-averaged ECGs were recorded during at exercise treadmill test at baseline, during exercise and during recovery.

---

## SUMMARY

For any ECG abnormality, always ask yourself:

*1. Could this be artefactual?*

If 'yes', consider:

- electrode misplacement
- external electrical interference
- incorrect calibration
- incorrect paper speed
- patient movement.

---

## FURTHER READING

Rajaganeshan R, Ludlam CL, Francis DP, *et al*. Accuracy in ECG lead placement among technicians, nurses, general physicians and cardiologists. *Int J Clin Pract* 2008; **62**: 65–70.

Samaniego NC, Morris F, Brady WJ. Electrocardiographic artefact mimicking arrhythmic change on the ECG. *Emerg Med J* 2003; **20**: 356–357.

Srikureja W, Darbar D, Reeder GS. Tremor-induced ECG artifact mimicking ventricular tachycardia. *Circulation* 2000; **102**: 1337–1338.

# Pacemakers and implantable cardioverter defibrillators

It is beyond the scope of this handbook to provide a detailed discussion of pacemakers and implantable cardioverter defibrillators (ICDs). However, we have included a brief overview in this chapter for two reasons:

- pacemakers and ICDs are effective treatments for several of the problems described in this book
- pacing affects the appearance of the ECG.

On the following pages you will find a general description of what pacemakers and ICDs do, along with their indications.

## WHAT DO PACEMAKERS DO?

Rapid advances in pacemaker technology have led to a remarkable increase in pacemaker sophistication, such that a wide range of different functions is now available. The most basic function of a pacemaker is to provide a 'safety net' for patients at risk of bradycardia. However, pacemakers that can terminate tachycardias and restore the synchronization of right and left ventricular contraction in heart failure are also available.

Pacemakers can be:

- **temporary** – a transvenous, transcutaneous or (rarely) transoesophageal pacing electrode is connected to an external pacemaker. This can provide pacing in an emergency, or tide patients over a short period of bradycardia (e.g. during a myocardial infarction) or until a permanent pacemaker can be implanted.
- **permanent** – the battery, electronics and electrode(s) are all implanted within the patient.

Patients seldom need pacing all the time, so both temporary and permanent pacemakers can be set up to monitor the heart's activity and provide impulses only when necessary. In the case of permanent pacemakers, this is an effective way of prolonging the lifetime of the battery, typically to between 7 and 15 years.

---

### PERCUSSION PACING

Cardiac pacing can sometimes be achieved with no mechanical aids whatsoever. First described in the 1960s, the technique of percussion pacing can help to stimulate QRS complexes to maintain a good cardiac output in a bradycardic patient. It is considerably less traumatic than chest compression. Percussion pacing is performed by delivering gentle blows to the precordium (alongside the lower left sternal edge) – the technique can be remarkably effective and can buy enough time to arrange further treatment as appropriate.

---

## INDICATIONS FOR TEMPORARY PACING

### Patients awaiting permanent pacing

If a patient has a severely symptomatic bradycardia but permanent pacing cannot be undertaken within an acceptable time, temporary pacing may be used to support them in the interim.

### Acute myocardial infarction

In acute **inferior** myocardial infarction, damage to the artery that supplies the atrio-ventricular (AV) node can cause complete heart block and bradycardia. Few patients need help with temporary pacing, as blood pressure is usually maintained despite the slow heart rate. Temporary pacing is needed in second-degree and third-degree AV block with symptoms or haemodynamic disturbance.

Acute **anterior** myocardial infarction often causes hypotension as a result of damage to the left ventricle. Extensive infarction may involve the bundle branches in the interventricular septum and cause bradycardia. Mortality is high. Temporary pacing is necessary for second-degree and third-degree AV block, even when the condition is asymptomatic.

### Tachycardia

Some tachycardias (e.g. ventricular tachycardia) can be terminated by **overdrive pacing**. This should only be undertaken under the guidance of someone experienced in the technique – contact a cardiologist for assistance.

### Perioperative pacing

See page 213 for further information.

## TEMPORARY PACEMAKER INSERTION AND CARE

Once the decision to insert a temporary transvenous pacemaker has been made, ensure that:

- the pacing wire is inserted by a trained member of staff using aseptic technique
- X-ray screening time is kept to a minimum
- a 'breathable' dressing is applied to the wound
- a chest radiograph is requested (and looked at!) after the pacemaker has been inserted to check for pneumothorax
- the function of the pacemaker is monitored daily by checking the pacing threshold and ensuring the output is set at double the threshold
- the pacing wire does not dislodge
- the pacing wire is removed at the earliest opportunity to prevent infection
- the pacing wire is replaced, if still required, after 5 days, after which time the risk of infection increases sharply
- temporary pacing is not withheld in acute myocardial infarction because of thrombolysis (the external jugular or femoral veins can be used for intravenous access routes in these circumstances, as these are superficial and easily compressed to control bleeding).

## INDICATIONS FOR PERMANENT PACING

The decision to implant a *permanent* pacemaker must be made by a cardiologist, and you should seek their advice if you are uncertain about referring a patient. Generally speaking, the following are indications for a permanent pacemaker:

- **Third-degree AV block** if chronic and symptomatic (class I indication). Most authorities would also support pacing in asymptomatic patients with acquired third-degree AV block (class IIa indication).
- **Second-degree AV block**, regardless of whether it is Mobitz type I or II, if chronic and symptomatic (class I indication). European guidelines would also support pacing for acquired asymptomatic second-degree AV block (Mobitz type I or II) as a class IIa indication. However, American guidelines advise against permanent pacemaker implantation for asymptomatic Mobitz type I second-degree AV block at the AV node level (or which is not known to be intra- or infra-Hisian) (class III indication).
- **Third-** or **second-degree AV block** after catheter ablation of the AV junction, or following valve surgery (if the block is not expected to resolve).
- **Third-** or **second-degree AV block** in the setting of a neuromuscular disease (e.g. myotonic muscular dystrophy).
- **Bifascicular** or **trifascicular block** with a clear history of syncope, or documented intermittent failure of the remaining fascicle.
- **Sinus node disease** causing symptomatic bradycardia. Pacing is not usually necessary for patients with no symptoms.
- **Malignant vasovagal syndrome** is helped by pacing only if it is of the 'cardio-inhibitory' variety that causes a bradycardia.
- **Carotid sinus syndrome** is also only helped by pacing when it is of the cardio-inhibitory variety associated with a bradycardia.

## SELECTION OF A PERMANENT PACEMAKER

A wide choice of permanent pacemakers is now available, each offering a different pacing strategy. The cardiologist will be responsible for selecting the most appropriate type of unit to be inserted, as well as for providing long-term follow-up.

There is an internationally accepted code of up to five letters to describe the type of pacemaker. Each letter describes an aspect of the pacemaker's function (see Table 20.1).

The following are some of the most commonly encountered pacemakers:

- **VVI**: this pacemaker has a single lead that senses activity in the ventricle. If no activity is detected, the pacemaker will take over control of the rhythm by pacing the ventricle via the same lead.
- **AAI**: this pacemaker also has a single lead, which is implanted in the atrium. It monitors atrial (P wave) activity. If normal atrial activity is not detected, it takes over by pacing the atria.
- **DDD**: this system has leads in both the atrium and the ventricle ('dual chamber'). It can both sense and pace via either lead. If it senses atrial activity but no ventricular activity, it will start pacing the ventricles in sequence with the atria.

**Table 20.1** Pacemaker codes

| Letter no. | Refers to | Code | Meaning |
| --- | --- | --- | --- |
| 1 | Chamber(s) paced | A | Atrium |
| | | V | Ventricle |
| | | D | Dual (both chambers) |
| 2 | Chamber(s) sensed | A | Atrium |
| | | V | Ventricle |
| | | D | Dual (both chambers) |
| | | O | None |
| 3 | Response to sensing | I | Inhibition of pacemaker |
| | | T | Triggering of pacemaker |
| | | D | Inhibition or triggering |
| | | O | None |
| 4 | Rate response | R | Rate-responsive pacemaker |
| 5 | Anti-tachycardia functions | P | Pacing of tachycardias |
| | | S | Shock delivered |
| | | D | Dual (pacing and shock) |
| | | O | None |

It can also pace the atria alone or, if AV conduction is blocked, pace the atria and ventricles sequentially.

- **AAIR, VVIR** and **DDDR**: the 'R' indicates that the pacemaker is rate responsive (see box below).

---

RATE RESPONSIVE PACEMAKER

A rate-responsive pacemaker adjusts its pacing rate according to the patient's level of activity to mimic the physiological response to exercise. Several parameters can be monitored by pacemakers to determine the patient's level of activity, including vibration, respiration and blood temperature.

---

## PACING AND THE ECG

Pacemakers activate depolarization with electrical impulses, and these appear as pacing 'spikes' on the ECG (Fig. 20.1). In ventricular pacing, a pacing spike will be followed by a broad QRS complex (because, arising from the ventricular myocardium, the impulse is conducted myocyte to myocyte rather than by the normal, fast-conduction pathways).

When the atria are being paced via an atrial lead, the pacing spike will be followed by a P wave. This may be conducted normally via the AV junction and followed by a normal QRS complex (Fig. 20.2). Alternatively, in dual-chamber sequential pacing, the P wave will be followed by a pacing spike from the ventricular lead and a broad QRS complex (Fig. 20.3).

Failure of a pacing spike to be followed by depolarization indicates a problem with 'capture', and a cardiologist should be contacted to arrange a pacemaker check.

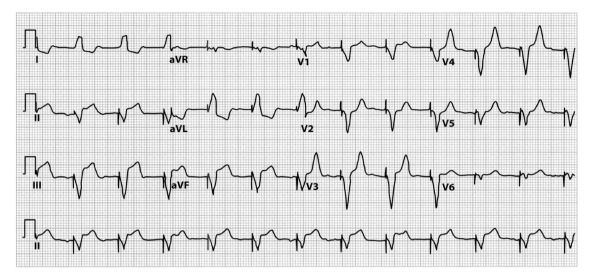

**Figure 20.1** Ventricular pacing.

Key point:    • Ventricular pacing spikes are followed by broad QRS complexes.

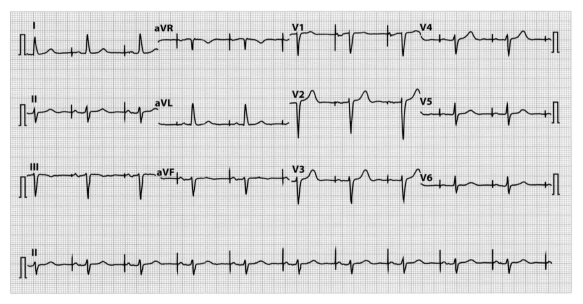

**Figure 20.2** Atrial pacing.

Key points:    • Atrial pacing spikes are followed by P waves.
                • There is normal atrioventricular conduction, so the QRS complexes are narrow.

## PACEMAKERS AND SURGERY

Pacemakers are relevant in surgery for two reasons:

• permanent pacemakers and diathermy
• temporary prophylactic perioperative pacing.

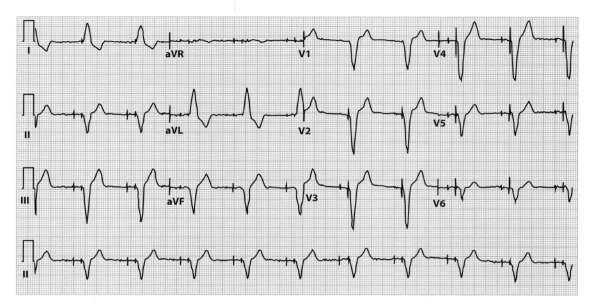

**Figure 20.3** Dual-chamber sequential pacing.

Key points:
- Atrial pacing spikes (small) are followed by P waves.
- Ventricular pacing spikes (large) are followed by broad QRS complexes.

Surgeons and anaesthetists must always be made aware if a patient undergoing surgery has a permanent pacemaker. Always ascertain the pacemaker type (patients usually carry an identification card with the pacemaker code on it) and the original indication for its insertion. It may also be advisable to arrange a check of the pacemaker before and after surgery.

Particular care must be taken during the operation to avoid interference with, or damage to, the pacemaker from diathermy. A particular risk of diathermy is that of inappropriate pacemaker inhibition, causing bradycardia or even asystole; it is therefore important to monitor the patient's ventricular rate closely throughout the procedure. To minimize the dangers, the 'active' diathermy electrode should be placed at least 15 cm from the pacemaker's generator box, and the 'indifferent' electrode as far from the box as possible.

Patients with certain cardiac conduction disorders who do *not* have a permanent pacemaker should be considered for a temporary pacemaker if they are about to undergo a procedure under general anaesthesia. Temporary pacing is indicated in:

- bradycardia with haemodynamic compromise
- third-degree AV block
- second-degree AV block.

Pacing is not usually necessary for bifascicular block unless the patient has a history of presyncope or syncope. Consult a cardiologist for further guidance.

## IMPLANTABLE CARDIOVERTER DEFIBRILLATORS

ICDs have proved to be invaluable in the management of life-threatening ventricular arrhythmias. Only a little larger than permanent pacemakers, they are implanted subcutaneously, usually in the same location as permanent pacemakers, although some of the older, bigger, units were implanted abdominally.

ICDs continually monitor the cardiac rhythm looking for ventricular arrhythmias. If an episode of ventricular tachycardia occurs, the device will normally begin by trying to overdrive pace the arrhythmia to terminate it. If that fails, the device will usually go on to deliver a shock. If ventricular fibrillation is detected, a shock is delivered as first-line treatment. The parameters by which ICDs diagnose arrhythmias and respond to them can be individually programmed into the device after it has been implanted, so that treatments most appropriate to the patient's condition can be chosen.

ICDs are expensive (costing £10,000–15,000) but effective, and many trials have shown marked reduction in mortality. According to the UK's National Institute for Health and Clinical Excellence, ICDs are indicated for 'secondary prevention' in patients who, in the absence of a treatable cause:

- have survived a cardiac arrest due to ventricular tachycardia or fibrillation
- have experienced spontaneous sustained ventricular tachycardia causing syncope or significant haemodynamic compromise
- have experienced spontaneous sustained ventricular tachycardia with a low left ventricular ejection fraction (<35%) and with heart failure symptoms no worse than New York Heart Association functional class III.

ICDs are indicated for 'primary prevention' in patients who have a history of previous myocardial infarction (at least four weeks ago) plus:
either

- a low left ventricular ejection fraction (<35%) and with heart failure symptoms no worse than New York Heart Association functional class III, plus non-sustained ventricular tachycardia on ambulatory ECG monitoring and inducible ventricular tachycardia on electrophysiological testing

or

- a low left ventricular ejection fraction (<30%) and with heart failure symptoms no worse than New York Heart Association functional class III, plus a QRS duration ≥120 ms.

ICDs should also be considered for 'primary prevention' in patients who have a history of a familial cardiac condition with a high risk of sudden death, such as:

- long QT syndrome
- hypertrophic cardiomyopathy
- Brugada syndrome
- arrhythmogenic right ventricular dysplasia (ARVD)

or who have undergone surgical repair of congenital heart disease.

## CARDIAC RESYNCHRONIZATION THERAPY (BIVENTRICULAR PACING)

In some patients with heart failure, the right and left ventricles do not contract simultaneously due to inter- and intra-ventricular conduction delays. This can impair left ventricular contractility, making symptoms of heart failure worse.

Pacing both the left and the right ventricles can restore synchronization of ventricular contraction, leading to improvements in quality of life and exercise tolerance, reduced mortality and reduced need for hospitalization in up to two-thirds of patients.

Cardiac resynchronization therapy is indicated in patients with advanced heart failure (left ventricular ejection fraction ≤35% and New York Heart Association functional class III or IV symptoms, on optimal drug therapy) and who are in sinus rhythm with either a QRS duration of ≥150 ms or a QRS duration of 120–149 ms and mechanical dyssynchrony on echocardiography.

Where a patient meets the criteria both for cardiac resynchronization therapy and an ICD (see above), a combined device (known as a CRT-D device) can be implanted.

## FURTHER READING

Epstein AE, DiMarco JP, Ellenbogen KA, *et al.* ACC/AHA/HRS 2008 guidelines for device-based therapy of cardiac rhythm abnormalities. A Report of the American College of Cardiology/American Heart Association task force on practice guidelines (writing committee to revise the ACC/AHA/NASPE 2002 guideline update for implantation of cardiac pacemakers and antiarrhythmia devices). *J Am Coll Cardiol* 2008; **51**: e1–62.

NICE Guideline TA95 – Implantable cardioverter defibrillators. Available for download from: http://guidance.nice.org.uk/TA95

NICE Guideline TA120 – Cardiac resynchronisation. Available for download from: http://guidance.nice.org.uk/TA120

Sutton R. Mobitz type 1 second degree atrioventricular block: the value of permanent pacing in the older patient. *Heart* 2013; **99**: 291–292.

Vardas PE, Auricchio A, Blanc JJ, *et al.* Guidelines for cardiac pacing and cardiac resynchronization therapy. The Task Force for Cardiac Pacing and Cardiac Resynchronization Therapy of the European Society of Cardiology. Developed in collaboration with the European Heart Rhythm Association. *Eur Heart J* 2007; **28**: 2256–2295.

20 Pacemakers and implantable cardioverter defibrillators

# CHAPTER 21

# Ambulatory ECG recording

The ECG is a key investigation in patients with palpitation, and may also be useful in patients with dizziness or syncope. However, most patients who complain of such symptoms only experience them intermittently. One of the limitations of the 12-lead ECG is that, in patients with a history of intermittent symptoms, the ECG is often entirely normal between episodes.

Although a 12-lead ECG recorded while the patient is asymptomatic might indicate the probable nature of an arrhythmia (for instance, the finding of a short PR interval makes atrioventricular re-entry tachycardia a likely diagnosis, whereas a long QT interval makes ventricular tachycardia (VT) more likely), there is no substitute for obtaining an ECG recording **during** a symptomatic episode. There are six ways in which this can be achieved:

- 24-h ambulatory ECG recording
- event recorder
- ECG 'on demand'
- bedside monitoring/telemetry (inpatient)
- implantable loop recorder
- external loop recorder.

Table 21.1 provides a guide to which modality of investigation is most useful in capturing an ECG during a symptomatic episode, depending on the frequency of the patient's symptoms.

**Table 21.1** Usefulness for capturing an ECG during an episode of palpitation

| Investigation method | Period between episodes | | |
|---|---|---|---|
| | Days | Weeks | Months |
| 24-h ambulatory ECG recording | +++ | + | + |
| Event recorder | +++ | ++ | + |
| ECG 'on demand' | +++* | +++* | +++* |
| Bedside monitoring/telemetry (inpatient) | +++ | + | + |
| Implantable loop recorder (ILR) | +++ | +++ | +++ |
| External loop recorder (ELR) | +++ | +++ | ++ |

+++ good; ++ fair; + poor.
*Only helpful if the patient is able to obtain an ECG during a symptomatic episode.

## 24-H AMBULATORY ECG RECORDING

The 24-h ambulatory ECG recording (Holter monitor) is one of the most frequently requested investigations in the assessment of patients with a suspected intermittent arrhythmia. The recorder is carried by the patient on a strap or belt and records the ECG via a small number of electrodes applied to the skin. The recording is usually made digitally onto a flash memory card. After the device is returned, the recording is analysed using appropriate software, looking for any rhythm disturbance.

One of the main drawbacks of the 24-h ambulatory ECG recorder is its short duration. Although recordings can take place over 48 h or even longer, the recording is usually only of value if the patient happens to experience an episode of palpitation, dizziness or syncope while wearing it. If a patient's symptoms are occurring on a daily basis, or two or three times a week, there is a reasonable probability of capturing an ECG during a symptomatic episode. With less frequent symptoms, the 24-h ambulatory ECG recording is much less likely to be informative.

Patients with intermittent symptoms are often reassured if their 24-h ECG recording was normal. However, such reassurance cannot be given if the patient was asymptomatic during the recording. This kind of false reassurance is a cause of great concern, as even patients with life-threatening arrhythmias may well have entirely normal ECG recordings between events. The key question to ask any patient about their 24-h ECG recording is: 'Did you experience your typical symptoms during the recording?' If the answer is 'No', the recording should be regarded as non-diagnostic and further investigation may need to be arranged.

Patients should always keep a symptom diary during the recording to help their recollection of events, and should be asked to note the exact time that any events occurred. During analysis of the recording, particular attention must be paid to those periods of the recording during which symptoms occurred, to allow accurate correlation between the symptoms experienced by the patient and their cardiac rhythm at the time.

## EVENT RECORDER

Event recorders are usually carried by the patient for longer periods than 24-h or 48-h ambulatory ECG recorders, the main difference being that they are used only to record the ECG during symptomatic episodes rather than continuously. To use an event recorder, the patient must be able to activate the device whenever symptoms occur – a recording is then obtained for a pre-determined duration (often around 30 s). With some devices, the patient can then transmit the recording back to the hospital by telephone for an immediate analysis of the cardiac rhythm.

There are two main types of event recorder: those that are continuously attached to the patient via ECG electrodes, and those that are only applied to the chest during an episode of palpitation. The former type is really just an extension of 24-h ambulatory ECG recording, the main difference being that the ECG is not recorded continuously, but instead is only recorded for a short period whenever the patient activates the device. Practical considerations (such as washing and skin irritation from the electrodes) mean that patients can usually only wear this type of event recorder for 7 days. The latter type is usually a small device that can be carried in the patient's pocket for as long as required. The device is held against the skin (usually over the anterior chest wall) and activated whenever symptoms occur.

Patients with relatively infrequent symptoms (occurring, for instance, on a weekly rather than a daily basis) can carry an event recorder in the hope of obtaining an ECG recording during a typical symptomatic episode. If the symptoms are less frequent (e.g. occurring every few months), an event recorder is unlikely to be helpful.

## ECG 'ON DEMAND'

In principle, one of the most effective ways to obtain an ECG recording during an episode of palpitation is to ask the patient to attend for an urgent ECG as soon as they notice the onset of symptoms. Practically, however, this approach poses a number of difficulties:

- the symptoms may not last long enough to give the patient time to reach a facility with an ECG machine
- the patient may not have transport available and it may be inadvisable for them to drive or to travel unaccompanied while symptomatic
- the patient may be asked to wait in line for an ECG when they arrive, by which time their symptoms may have resolved.

Nonetheless, this can be a rewarding approach, particularly if a patient's symptoms are relatively mild and infrequent (e.g. only occurring every few weeks or months) but last for long enough for them to reach a facility with an ECG machine. The patient should be given a form or letter (see box) and advised to take it to their nearest general practitioner or hospital emergency department (or ECG department) when they develop symptoms. The letter should be on official notepaper and should request that whoever sees the patient must perform a 12-lead ECG **as soon as possible** if the patient presents with symptoms. The letter should also give an address to which a copy of the ECG should be sent **and**, in case the ECG goes astray, should ask that the patient also be given a copy to keep. The patient should then bring any ECGs recorded in this way to their next consultation.

---

### SUGGESTED LETTER FORMAT FOR ECG 'ON DEMAND'

To Whom It May Concern

Re: [insert patient's details here]

The above-named patient is currently undergoing investigation for palpitation. The patient has been instructed to try to obtain a 12-lead ECG if they experience a symptomatic episode.

If the patient presents to you with palpitation, please would you obtain a good-quality 12-lead ECG recording as rapidly as possible (before the symptoms resolve). Please write on the ECG recording whether the patient's symptoms were still present at the time of the recording.

I would be grateful if you would send a copy of the ECG to [insert doctor's details here]. Please also give a copy to the patient to bring to their next consultation.

Thank you.

[Insert name and signature here]

---

## BEDSIDE MONITORING/TELEMETRY (INPATIENT)

If the symptoms are frequent (e.g. daily) and sufficiently troublesome to merit an urgent diagnosis, one option that is likely to yield a diagnosis is to admit the patient to hospital and use a bedside cardiac monitor (or telemetry). The patient should be instructed to inform the nursing staff immediately whenever he or she experiences symptoms so that the monitor can be checked and a recording obtained. Many bedside ECG monitors now incorporate diagnostic software that is sophisticated enough to detect most (but not all) significant arrhythmias, sound an alarm and store (or print out) a rhythm strip.

This approach can be effective at obtaining a diagnosis, but its limitations are that it can be expensive, it can be inconvenient for patients and it takes patients out of their 'everyday' environment and activities, which might affect the frequency of their symptoms.

## IMPLANTABLE LOOP RECORDER (ILR)

The patient who experiences severe but infrequent symptoms, such as unheralded syncope occurring once every few months, presents one of the most challenging problems. In this case the urgent need to identify a potentially dangerous rhythm disturbance (such as VT or intermittent third-degree atrioventricular block) is made more difficult by its infrequent occurrence. Even an event recorder is a rather hit-and-miss method of capturing symptomatic episodes and, if the patient loses consciousness, they may not be able to activate a recorder until after the rhythm disturbance has resolved and they have regained consciousness.

An ILR device (such as Medtronic's Reveal® DX and Reveal® XT devices) provides a useful means of attempting to capture an ECG during one of these infrequent episodes. The ILR device is small (and has no attached leads) and is implanted subcutaneously in a similar position to a permanent pacemaker. It contains a battery (which lasts up to three years) and a digital recorder that monitors the ECG and records a rhythm strip. The ILR works on a loop principle, so that the earliest rhythm recording is continuously overwritten by the latest on a continuous 'rolling' basis. The amount of storage available varies according to the device and its settings.

If an event occurs, the recording loop can be 'frozen' by the patient using an activation device that is held against the recorder ('patient activation'). ILRs also contain diagnostic software that can be programmed to identify and store asymptomatic rhythm disturbances ('auto activation'). The recordings can then be downloaded at a later date by the centre where the ILR was implanted. There is sufficient memory in the ILR to record several loops before a download is necessary.

The ILR represents a useful way to record the ECG in those patients whose symptoms are infrequent but nonetheless worrying. Its usefulness has to be weighed against the need for an invasive procedure (with the associated risks of scarring and infection) and the cost of the device, although the cost is somewhat offset by the reduced need for multiple non-invasive ambulatory recordings.

## EXTERNAL LOOP RECORDER (ELR)

A non-invasive alternative to the ILR is an ELR (e.g. Sorin SpiderFlash-t™), a loop recorder that is worn externally. Like the ILR, the ELR works on a loop principle, such that the ECG is recorded continuously and the last few minutes is always held in memory before being overwritten with new data. Because they have to be worn externally, they're not as practical as ILRs for very long-term monitoring. However they can provide monitoring over a period of weeks, and this may be long enough to allow a good chance to capture a symptomatic event.

# FURTHER READING

Brignole M, Vardas P, Hoffman E, *et al*. Indications for the use of diagnostic implantable and external ECG loop recorders. *Europace* 2009; **11**: 671–687.

Crawford MH, Bernstein SJ, Deedwania PC, *et al*. ACC/AHA Guidelines for ambulatory electrocardiography: executive summary and recommendations. A report of the American College of Cardiology/American Heart Association task force on practice guidelines (committee to revise the guidelines for ambulatory electrocardiography) developed in collaboration with the North American Society for Pacing and Electrophysiology. *Circulation* 1999; **100**: 886–893.

Jabaudon D, Sztajzel J, Sievert K, *et al*. Usefulness of ambulatory 7-day ECG monitoring for the detection of atrial fibrillation and flutter after acute stroke and transient ischemic attack. *Stroke* 2004; **35**: 1647–1651.

Kala R, Viitasalo MT, Toivonen L, *et al*. Ambulatory ECG recording in patients referred because of syncope or dizziness. *Acta Med Scand Suppl* 1982; **668**: 13–19.

NICE Guideline CG109 – Transient loss of consciousness in adults and young people. Available for download from: http://guidance.nice.org.uk/CG109

# CHAPTER 22

# Exercise ECG testing

The symptom-limited exercise ECG can be a valuable tool for the assessment of patients with ischaemic heart disease and exercise-related arrhythmias. However, failure to interpret exercise ECGs correctly limits their usefulness.

In this chapter, we will help you to answer the following questions:

- What are the indications for an exercise ECG?
- What are the risks of an exercise ECG?
- How do I perform an exercise ECG?
- When do I stop an exercise ECG?
- How do I interpret an exercise ECG?

## WHAT ARE THE INDICATIONS FOR AN EXERCISE ECG?

Exercise ECG testing can be useful in:

- assessing cardiopulmonary fitness
- investigating exertional dyspnoea
- risk stratification in stable angina
- risk stratification after myocardial infarction
- assessing exercise-induced arrhythmias
- assessing the need for a permanent pacemaker
- assessing exercise tolerance
- assessing response to treatment.

Exercise ECG testing should always be undertaken with a specific question in mind, and an appreciation of its limitations. In particular, it should only be performed if the information you are likely to gain outweighs the potential (albeit small) risks.

> ### EXERCISE ECG TESTING IN CORONARY ARTERY DISEASE
>
> Although exercise ECG testing can be useful in the assessment of patients with known coronary artery disease, it should not be used to diagnose or exclude stable angina in patients who are not already known to have coronary artery disease. Despite the frequent use of exercise ECG testing in this context historically, the diagnostic value of exercise ECG testing for the *de novo* diagnosis or exclusion of coronary artery disease is poor compared with other available tests. The diagnosis of stable angina should therefore be based upon clinical history and cardiovascular risk factors, supplemented where necessary by functional or anatomical imaging, as outlined by the NICE guideline on chest pain of recent onset (see *Further Reading*).

# WHAT ARE THE RISKS OF AN EXERCISE ECG?

As with all procedures, exercise ECG testing carries risks:

- morbidity of 2.4 in 10,000
- mortality of 1 in 10,000 (within 1 week of testing).

To minimize the risks, always take a patient history and perform an examination to check for **absolute** contraindications to exercise ECG testing (Table 22.1).

In addition, there are several **relative** contraindications to exercise testing, in the presence of which the test should only be performed with a full awareness of the increased risks involved and under close medical supervision (Table 22.2).

**Table 22.1** Absolute contraindications to an exercise ECG

- Recent myocardial infarction (within 7 days)
- Unstable angina (rest pain within previous 48 h)
- Severe aortic stenosis or hypertrophic obstructive cardiomyopathy
- Acute myocarditis
- Acute pericarditis
- Uncontrolled hypertension
  - systolic BP >250 mmHg
  - diastolic BP >120 mmHg
- Uncontrolled heart failure
- Recent thromboembolic episode (pulmonary or systemic)
- Acute febrile illness

**Table 22.2** Relative contraindications to an exercise ECG

- Recent myocardial infarction (within 7 days to 1 month)*
- Known severe coronary artery disease
- Known serious risk of arrhythmia
- Mild or moderate aortic stenosis or hypertrophic obstructive cardiomyopathy
- Pulmonary hypertension
- Significant left ventricular dysfunction
- Aneurysm (ventricular or aortic)
- Highly abnormal resting ECG
  - left or right bundle branch block
  - digoxin effect
- Frail patients

*A submaximal exercise test should be used.

# HOW DO I PERFORM AN EXERCISE ECG?

Unless the exercise test is being performed to assess the effectiveness of treatment, patients should be advised to tail-off any existing anti-anginal treatment over the 3 days before the test. They can use sublingual glyceryl trinitrate until 1 h before the test.

On the day of the test, ensure that two people trained in cardiopulmonary resuscitation (CPR) are present for supervision and that all the necessary drugs and

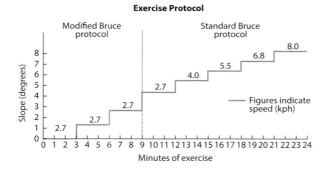

**Figure 22.1** The Bruce and modified Bruce protocols.

| Protocol | Modified Bruce | | | Standard Bruce | | | | |
|---|---|---|---|---|---|---|---|---|
| Stage | 01 | 02 | 03 | 1 | 2 | 3 | 4 | 5 |
| Speed (kph) | 2.7 | 2.7 | 2.7 | 2.7 | 4.0 | 5.5 | 6.8 | 8.0 |
| Slope (degrees) | 0 | 1.3 | 2.6 | 4.3 | 5.4 | 6.3 | 7.2 | 8.1 |

equipment for CPR are available. After explaining the test to the patient and checking for contraindications (see previous section), decide which exercise protocol to use. There are many different protocols, but the two most commonly used are:

● the Bruce protocol
● the modified Bruce protocol.

The modified Bruce protocol begins with a lighter workload than the Bruce protocol, and is particularly suitable for frail patients or those being assessed after a recent myocardial infarction (Fig. 22.1).

After reviewing the patient's resting ECG and checking their blood pressure, they can commence exercise. Monitor their symptoms and ECG throughout, and check their blood pressure every 3 min. Reasons for stopping the test are discussed below.

After the completion of exercise, continue to monitor the patient's ECG and blood pressure until any symptoms or ECG changes have fully resolved.

> **WHAT IS A MET?**
>
> The workload at each level of an exercise protocol can be expressed in terms of metabolic equivalents (or METs). One MET, the rate of oxygen consumption by a normal person at rest, is 3.5 mL/kg per min. To perform the activities of daily living requires 5 METs.

## WHEN DO I STOP AN EXERCISE ECG?

One indicator of a good prognosis is the ability to achieve a target heart rate with no symptoms or major ECG changes. The target heart rate is calculated as follows:

● target heart rate = 220 minus patient's age (in years)

However, several events may require the exercise test to be stopped before the target heart rate is reached. The test *must* be stopped if:

● the patient asks for the test to be stopped

- the systolic blood pressure falls by >20 mmHg
- the heart rate falls by >10 beats/min
- the patient develops >4 mm ST segment depression with chest pain
- sustained ventricular or supraventricular arrhythmias occur.

In addition, consider stopping the test if the patient develops:

- >2 mm ST segment depression and chest pain
- >3 mm asymptomatic ST segment depression
- >1 mm ST segment elevation
- conduction disturbance and chest pain
- non-sustained ventricular tachycardia
- systolic blood pressure >250 mmHg or diastolic >150 mmHg
- dizziness
- marked or disproportionate breathlessness
- severe fatigue or exhaustion.

## HOW DO I INTERPRET AN EXERCISE ECG?

If the exercise ECG was done to induce an exercise-related arrhythmia, it should be fairly clear whether the test has succeeded in doing so. The interpretation of arrhythmias is the subject of the earlier chapters in this book. Repeating the exercise test once the patient has been established on treatment can be helpful in assessing its efficacy.

The most common indicator of myocardial ischaemia on exercise ECG testing is the development of ST segment depression. However, care must be taken when measuring ST segment depression during exercise, as depression of the **J point** (the junction of the S wave and ST segment) is normal. The ST segment slopes upwards sharply after the J point, and returns to the baseline within 60 ms (1.5 small squares). Therefore, measure ST segment depression **80 ms (2 small squares) beyond the J point** (Fig. 22.2).

ST segment depression is not the only noteworthy result, however. T wave inversion may develop during exercise, as may bundle branch block, although these can occur without major coronary artery disease. A fall in systolic blood pressure often indicates severe coronary artery disease.

The 12-lead ECG in Figure 22.3 shows anterolateral horizontal ST segment depression in the early recovery period, immediately after completing 3 minutes and 51 seconds of exercise, in a patient with known coronary artery disease. Figure 22.4

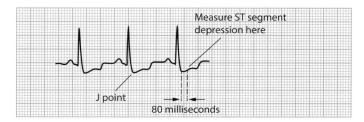

**Figure 22.2** The J point.

Key points:
- The J point is the junction of the S wave and ST segment.
- Measure ST segment depression 80 ms after the J point.

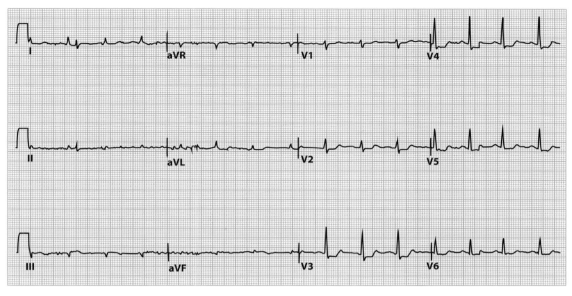

**Figure 22.3** Exercise ECG test in a patient with coronary artery disease.

Key point:    • This ECG was recorded in the early recovery period. There is anterolateral ST segment depression.

shows the accompanying signal-averaged ECGs across all 12 leads, as measured at baseline, after 2 minutes and 10 seconds, at peak exercise (3 minutes and 51 seconds), and during the recovery period. The vertical markers on each ECG identify the start and end of the QRS complex and the J point.

When reporting an exercise ECG, include the following information:

- the patient's identifying details
- the date and time of the test
- why the test was performed
- a list of the patient's medication, highlighting anything omitted prior to the test
- a description of the baseline (resting) 12-lead ECG
- total exercise and recovery time
- resting and peak heart rate
- resting and peak blood pressure
- calculated target heart rate and whether this was attained
- total METs attained
- any symptoms that occurred, or whether the patient remained asymptomatic
- whether there was any ST segment depression
  - which leads were affected
  - horizontal, upsloping or downsloping
  - time of onset and time taken for subsequent normalization
  - maximum depth (mm), measured 80 ms beyond the J point
- any arrhythmias that occurred
- any other ECG changes (e.g. ST segment elevation, bundle branch block).

22 Exercise ECG testing

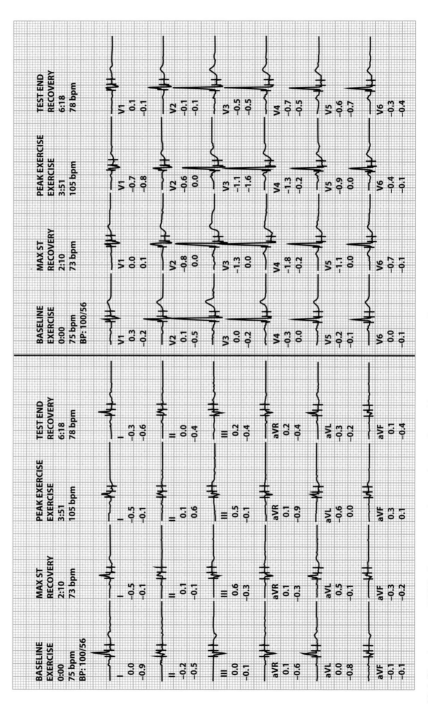

**Figure 22.4** Signal-averaged ECGs from an exercise test in a patient with coronary artery disease.

Key point    • There is anterolateral ST segment depression.

# FURTHER READING

Banerjee A, Newman DR, Van den Bruel A, *et al*. Diagnostic accuracy of exercise stress testing for coronary artery disease: a systematic review and meta-analysis of prospective studies. *Int J Clin Pract* 2012; **66**: 477–492.

Gibbons RJ, Balady GJ, Bricker JT, *et al*. ACC/AHA 2002 guideline update for exercise testing: summary article: a report of the American College of Cardiology/American Heart Association Task Force on Practice Guidelines (Committee to Update the 1997 Exercise Testing Guidelines). *Circulation* 2002; **106**: 1883–1892.

NICE guideline on chest pain of recent onset (2010). Downloadable from: http://guidance.nice.org.uk/CG95

Van der Wall EE. The exercise ECG: still a useful exercise? *Neth Heart J* 2009; **17**: 47.

# Appendix 1: ECG resources

## TEXTBOOKS

### General cardiology textbooks

Bonow RO, Mann DL, Zipes DP, Libby P (eds). *Braunwald's Heart Disease: A Textbook of Cardiovascular Medicine*, 9th edn. Philadelphia: Elsevier Health Sciences, 2011. ISBN-13: 978-1437727081.

Camm AJ, Lüscher TF, Serruys PW (eds). *The ESC Textbook of Cardiovascular Medicine,* 2nd edn. Oxford: Oxford University Press, 2009. ISBN-13: 978-0199566990.

Ramrakha P, Hill J. *Oxford Handbook of Cardiology,* 2nd edn. Oxford: Oxford University Press, 2012. ISBN-13: 978-0199643219.

### ECG interpretation

Huff J. *ECG Workout: Exercises in Arrhythmia Interpretation*, 6th edn. Philadelphia: Lippincott Williams & Wilkins, 2011. ISBN-13: 978-1451115536.

Jenkins D, Gerred S. *ECGs by Example*, 3rd edn. Edinburgh: Churchill Livingstone, 2011. ISBN-13: 978-0702042287.

Springhouse Publishing. *ECG interpretation Made Incredibly Easy!* 5th edn. Philadelphia: Lippincott Williams & Wilkins, 2010. ISBN-13: 978-1608312894.

### Electrophysiology & pacing

Bashir Y, Betts TR, Rajappan K. *Cardiac Electrophysiology and Catheter Ablation*. Oxford: Oxford University Press, 2010. ISBN-13: 978-0199550180.

Ramsdale DR, Rao A. *Cardiac Pacing and Device Therapy*. Berlin: Springer, 2012. ISBN-13: 978-1447129387.

Timperley J, Leeson P, Mitchell ARJ, Betts T. *Pacemakers and ICDs*. Oxford: Oxford University Press, 2007. ISBN-13: 978-0198571322.

## KEY GUIDELINES

Key guidance published by the Society for Cardiological Science and Technology (available from http://www.scst.org.uk):

- Recording a Standard 12-Lead Electrocardiogram
- Resting 12-Lead ECG Electrode Placement and Associated Problems.

Key guidance published by the American College of Cardiology (available from http://www.cardiosource.org) in partnership with its sister organizations: Recommendations for the Standardization and Interpretation of the Electrocardiogram:

Part 1 – The Electrocardiogram and Its Technology

Part 2 – Electrocardiography Diagnostic Statement List

Part 3 – Intraventricular Conduction Disturbances

Part 4 – The ST Segment, T and U Waves, and the QT Interval

Part 5 – Electrocardiogram Changes Associated with Cardiac Chamber Hypertrophy

Part 6 – Acute Ischaemia/Infarction

ACC/AHA Clinical Competence Statement on Electrocardiography and Ambulatory Electrocardiography

ACC Expert Consensus Document on Signal-Averaged Electrocardiography.

Corrado D, Pelliccia A, Heidbuchel H, *et al*. Recommendations for interpretation of 12-lead electrocardiogram in the athlete. *Eur Heart J* 2010; **31**; 243–259.

## SOCIETIES

Heart Rhythm UK
http://www.heartrhythmuk.org.uk/

European Cardiac Arrhythmia Society
http://www.ecas-heartrhythm.org/

European Heart Rhythm Association
http://www.escardio.org/communities/EHRA/Pages/welcome.aspx

Heart Rhythm Society
http://www.hrsonline.org/

## WEBSITES

The following websites are particularly useful for anyone wanting to learn more about ECG interpretation:

*ECGpedia*: http://en.ecgpedia.org/wiki/Main_Page

*ECG Learning Center*: http://ecg.utah.edu

*Skillstat ECG Simulator*: http://www.skillstat.com/tools/ecg-simulator

# Appendix 2: Help with the next edition

We would like to know what should be included (or omitted!) in the next edition of *Making Sense of the ECG*. Please write with your comments or suggestions to

Dr Andrew R. Houghton
Making Sense of the ECG
c/o CRC Press
The Taylor & Francis Group
2-4 Park Square
Milton Park
Abingdon
Oxfordshire
OX14 4RN
United Kingdom

We will acknowledge all suggestions that are used.

# Index